Vaccines in Developing Countries:
Needs, Production Capacity and Immunization Strategies

Vaccines in Developing Countries:

Needs, Production Capacity and Immunization Strategies

Editors

Mahmoud M. Bahgat

The National Research Centre and
Academy of Scientific Research and Technology,
Cairo, Egypt

Ibeh Bartholomew

National Biotechnology Development Agency,
Abuja, Nigeria

ALLIED PUBLISHERS PVT. LTD.

New Delhi • Mumbai • Kolkata • Chennai • Bangalore • Hyderabad

ALLIED PUBLISHERS PRIVATE LIMITED

1/13-14 Asaf Ali Road, **New Delhi**–110002
Ph.: 011-23239001 • E-mail: delhi.books@alliedpublishers.com

17 Chittaranjan Avenue, **Kolkata**–700072
Ph.: 033-22129618 • E-mail: cal.books@alliedpublishers.com

15 J.N. Heredia Marg, Ballard Estate, **Mumbai**–400001
Ph.: 022-42126969 • E-mail: mumbai.books@alliedpublishers.com

No. 25/10, Commander-in-Chief Road, Ethiraj Lane (Next to Post Office)
Egmore, **Chennai**–600008
Ph.: 044-28223938 • E-mail: chennai.books@alliedpublishers.com

P.B. No. 9932, 1st Floor, Sunkada Chickkana Complex, Loop Lane Off Race Course Road
Next to Hotel Maurya, Gandhi Nagar, **Bangalore**–560 009
Ph.: 080-22262081 • E-Mail: bngl.books@alliedpublishers.com

Sri Jayalakshmi Nilayam, No. 3-4-510, 3rd Floor (Above More Super Market)
Barkatpura, **Hyderabad**–500027
Ph.: 040-27551811, 040-27551812 • E-mail: hyd.books@alliedpublishers.com

Website: www.alliedpublishers.com

ISBN: 978-81-942903-3-9

Published by Sunil Sachdev and printed by Ravi Sachdev at Allied Publishers Pvt. Ltd.,
1/13-14 Asaf Ali Road, New Delhi–110002

Department of Biochemistry
University of Delhi South Campus
Benito Juarez Road, New Delhi–110021, India.
Tel: +91-11-24111967/24114159 (Office)
Fax: +91-11-24115270
Mobile: 9810696767
E-mail: dpsarkar59@gmail.com

Debi P. Sarkar
Ph.D, FAScT, FNASc, FASc, FNA
Professor & Former Dean, Former Director,
IISER Mohali, JC Bose National Fellow

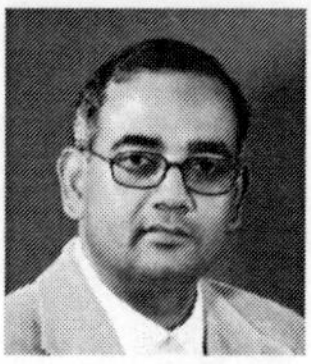

Foreword

NAM S&T Centre Publication
on
'Vaccines in Developing Countries: Needs, Production Capacity and Immunization Strategies'

Vaccines have long been used to combat various infectious diseases; however, the last decade has witnessed a revolution in the trends and approaches to vaccine design and development and vaccine sustainability practices. No longer is there a need to rely on the laborious conventional methods such as attenuation or killing the pathogens. Now sophisticated and advanced technologies such as DNA vaccines, recombinant vaccines and epitope-based, or peptide vaccines are used to stimulate the types of immune response. These genetic vaccines categorized as the third generation vaccines contain the DNA that codes for specific proteins (antigens) from a pathogen. The DNA is injected into the body and taken up by the cells, whose normal metabolic processes synthesize proteins based on the genetic code in the plasmid that they have taken up. Never has research in this area been more exciting.

I am pleased to learn that the Centre for Science and Technology of the Non-Aligned and Other Developing Countries (NAM S&T Centre) had organized an International Workshop on ***"Modern and Emerging Trend in Vaccine Development"*** during May 22–24, 2018 in Abuja, Nigeria in collaboration with the National Biotechnology Development Agency (NABDA), Abuja, Nigeria. The major objective of this Workshop was to provide a platform for brainstorming among the scientists, researchers, industry experts, academicians and other concerned professionals on the third generation vaccine development approaches i.e. DNA vaccination or genetic immunization which has greater efficacy and other potential advantages over the currently available conventional vaccines offering prevention against various infectious diseases.

As a follow up, the NAM S&T Centre has brought out this book which comprises 15 papers contributed by the participants of the Abuja Workshop. The volume has been edited by Prof. (Dr.) Mahmoud M. Bahgat, Professor of Biochemistry, The National Research Centre, Academy of Scientific Research and Technology, Cairo, Egypt and Dr. Ibeh Bartholomew, Acting Director and Head of Department of Medical Biotechnology, National Biotechnology Development Agency (NABDA), Abuja, Nigeria. The papers included in this book highlight the new and emerging research in vaccine development and immunization trends which are being followed in various developing countries including their transition status from the first to third generation vaccine development.

I congratulate the NAM S&T Centre for bringing out this valuable publication which will be of immense use to scientists, researchers and others engaged in revolutionizing the conventional approaches to vaccine design and development in basic and translational medicines for improved treatment of various emerging bacterial and viral diseases.

19th July 2019 **(Debi P. Sarkar)**

Introduction

The developing countries have witnessed the emergence of threats of several new infectious diseases over the past two decades as sporadic events almost every year. The recent outbreak of Ebola, SARS, Zika Virus reminds us how helpless we are in dealing with any such situations despite three decades of vaccine research. Vaccine development plays a very important role in combating the infectious diseases and despite the massive expansion in our understanding of immune responses, there is still a great need for new vaccines, which is occurring far more slowly than it should be. The reason for this slow pace of vaccine development has two different dimensions. On the one hand, we need to understand more about the identification of suitable antigens, adjuvants and delivery methods while on the other there are regulatory, technical and manufacturing hurdles. Even though the technologies today can provide adequate tools to detect, control and prevent the emerging infections, the developing countries are still suffering from a variety of infectious diseases for which either the suitable vaccines do not exist or need further research and development, requiring global collaboration and coordination among the regulatory agencies as well as sustainable economic system to support such initiatives.

Considering the global efforts in vaccine development and ever increasing challenges simultaneously, the international community needs to identify the current challenges. There are three core areas which need to be addressed, viz. (i) dealing with sizeable gaps in vaccine coverage around the world, (ii) developing new vaccines for serious infectious diseases such as HIV/AIDS, Hepatitis C, Tuberculosis and Malaria and (iii) Vaccines for non-communicable diseases like cancer, asthma and multiple sclerosis which are the major cause of morbidity and mortality worldwide.

The Global Vaccine Action Plan 2011–2020 (GVAP) of the World Health Organization (WHO) is dedicated to "Health and Well-Being", while addressing the three core areas of vaccine development mentioned above. The UN Sustainable Development Goal, SDG-3 particularly aims, among other things, to control AIDS, tuberculosis, malaria, and neglected tropical diseases and to reduce the premature mortality from non-communicable diseases to one third by 2030, as well as to combat hepatitis, water-borne diseases, and other communicable diseases. The GVAP further strengthen the routine immunization to meet vaccination coverage targets, and accelerate the control of vaccine-preventable diseases.

Keeping the above in view, the Centre for Science and Technology of the Non-Aligned and Other Developing Countries (NAM S&T Centre) in partnership with National Biotechnology Development Agency (NABDA), Abuja, Nigeria organized an International Workshop on '*Modern and Emerging Trend in Vaccine Development*' in Abuja, Nigeria, from 22–24 May 2018, which brought together 89 scientists, researchers and policy makers from 17 countries to address the challenges that many developing countries are facing in the area of vaccine design and development.

As a follow up of the Abuja International Workshop, the present book titled '***Vaccines in Developing Countries: Needs, Production Capacity and Immunization Strategies***' is being published by the NAM S&T Centre which includes 15 scientific and technical papers contributed by the experts/participants from 9 different countries.

I appreciate the efforts put in place by both of our Editors Prof. Mahmoud M. Bahgat from Egypt and Dr. Ibeh Bartholomew from Nigeria for the technical editing of the manuscripts. I also acknowledge the interest and valuable efforts of the entire team of NAM S&T Centre and am especially thankful to Mr. M. Bandyopadhyay, Dr. (Mrs.) Kavita Mehra, Ms. Jasmeet Kaur, Ms. Nidhi Utreja and Mr. Pankaj Buttan in compiling and proof reading of the manuscripts, liaising with authors, designing the cover page, formatting and taking all the necessary actions in giving a shape to this book.

A special thanks to Prof. Arun P. Kulshreshtha, Former Director-General of NAM S&T Centre, for his interest and support in organising this very important valuable event.

I am sure this book will be of immense use to all those associated with issues related to vaccine development.

(Amitava Bandopadhyay)
Director General
NAM S&T Centre

Preface

The UN has reaffirmed the global community's commitments towards poverty eradication, protecting environment and improving human health and well being in its 2030 Sustainable Development Goals. This can be achieved by building global partnerships and coalitions which closely and willingly work together to achieve such goals.

Infections fall amongst major environmental hazards which endanger human health and contribute to the increasing poverty worldwide. The control of infection is implemented through raising hygienic measures, availability of anti-infective drugs and development of new ones and most important, the availability of protective vaccines against various infections. Hygienic measures, if respected and seriously considered, can singly limit infections; nevertheless, this has never been hundred percent efficiently implemented worldwide.

Anti-infective drugs and/or therapies are available and can treat acute infections; however, they do not protect against re-infection. It suffices to say that both protective and therapeutic (prophylactic) vaccines are the best options to protect against new infections, re-infections or emerging infections and to minimize to the barest pathological consequences of past infections.

Vaccine development is a never ending story. It starts at the available technology and is always a subject for upgrading with the emergence of modern technologies. The trend can be clearly seen in the development of vaccines from killed or attenuated organisms to subunit protein vaccines and currently from DNA vaccines to reverse genetics based re-assorted viral vaccines. This means that research and development (R&D) is and will continue to be a major issue in revolutionizing the vaccination strategies.

In this book, we had for the first time a unique opportunity to review and summarize the vaccination strategies, R&D capacities, and vaccines production facilities in nine (9) of the forty-seven (47) member countries of the Centre for Science & Technology of the Non-Aligned and Other Developing Countries (NAM S&T Centre) including Egypt, India, Myanmar, Nepal, Nigeria, Palestine, Peru, Sri Lanka and Vietnam. The chapters included in this book are mainly the outcomes of the presentations made in the International Workshop on "*Modern and Emerging Trend in Vaccine Development*" that was organized in Abuja,

Nigeria on 22–24 May, 2018 by NAM S&T Centre, India and NABDA, Nigeria.

We believe that this book would tremendously contribute to any future action for controlling infections in the reported countries as it includes valuable knowledge on vaccination strategies against different infections. It also highlights the revolutionary technologies on improving vaccination efficacies and strategies. Readers from the developing nations would find it useful as the book summarizes vaccine usage in the NAM and other developing countries as well as review the history of establishment of some vaccine production capacities in these countries.

We hope that readers can make use of such documentation to build the needed networks and collaborations with the aim to lower incidence and prevalence of infections which will contribute to lowering poverty, protecting environment and improving human health and well being in the NAM countries and beyond.

Prof. (Dr.) Mahmoud M. Bahgat
The National Research Centre and Academy of Scientific Research and Technology, Cairo, Egypt

Dr. Ibeh Bartholomew
National Biotechnology Development Agency, Abuja, Nigeria

Contents

SECTION 1

Selected Country Vaccination Approach

Vaccines and Vaccination: Current Status and Future Challenges

Harish Padh[1] and Priti Desai[2]

[1]Sardar Patel University, Vallabh Vidhyanagar, Gujarat, India

[2]School of Biological Sciences and Biotechnology, Institute of Advanced Research, Koba, Gandhinagar, Gujarat, India

E-mail: [1]hpadh@yahoo.com

ABSTRACT: Vaccination has saved millions of lives ever since it was adopted at a larger scale guided by WHO and UNICEF as an Expanded Program of Immunization. Key hurdle now is to reach out to the remote areas in developing countries. The Global Vaccine Action Plan (GVAP) of the WHO (2011–2020) aims to achieve full vaccination coverage. Other challenging issues are the quality of supplied vaccines and conducting research to develop better vaccines to meet the unmet medical needs of today and tomorrow. Unfortunately, the effect of vaccination programs are seen after decades and hence, its impact is not immediately perceived, thus, it falls in lower priority in developing countries. With GVAP, it is hoped that the situation will improve.

Keywords: Public Health, Vaccination Coverage, Research, Newer Better Vaccines, GVAP, Vaccine Manufacturing, Developing Countries.

1. INTRODUCTION

Vaccine is a biological preparation that provides active acquired immunity to a particular disease. A vaccine typically contains an agent that resembles a disease-causing microorganism or some of its molecules, often made from weakened or killed microbes or its toxins or one of its distinctive antigens. The antigen activates the body's immune system to recognize the antigen as a threat and destroy it. This also enabled the immune system to recognize and destroy other microorganisms as well, associated with that antigen if it may encounter in the future by the same host. Perhaps over simplified but this process of vaccination has freed mankind from many fatal or devastating diseases like smallpox, plague and protected from several others.

1.1 History of Vaccination

In the eighteenth century small-pox killed around 10 percent of the population, with the number as high as 20 percent in towns and cities where infection spread more easily. In that era, the British Surgeon, Edward Jenner made a brilliant observation that milkmaids were generally immune to smallpox. He postulated that the pus in the blisters that milkmaids received from cowpox (a disease similar to smallpox, but much less virulent) protected them from smallpox, which in 1796 led to the first vaccine for smallpox. His work is said to have saved more lives than the work of any other human.

In the nineteenth century, vaccination nearly eliminated incidents of smallpox in the Western countries, but it was still prevalent in Africa and Asia during the first half of the twentieth century. The WHO launched its ***Intensified Smallpox Eradication Programme*** in 1967, and soon the disease had been wiped out globally. Such dramatic eradication of smallpox through vaccination resulted in the concept that a similar approach should be taken with other preventable diseases. Vaccination has now taken roots in the healthcare and medical world.

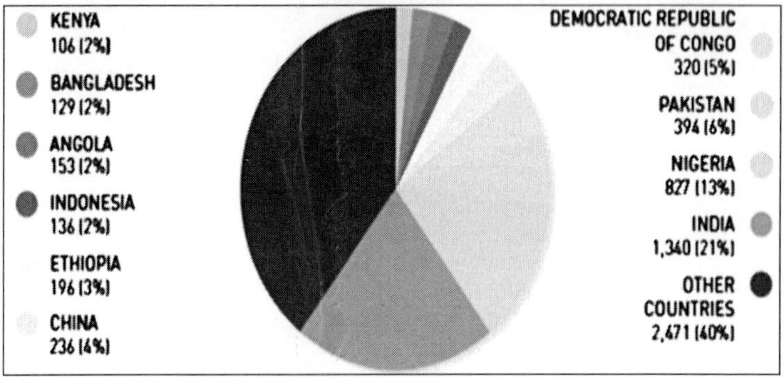

Fig. 1: *Infant Mortality Burden (IMB)* in Developing Economies, India Shares 21% of IMB which is very Alarming among the Developing Countries

(*Source:* GAVI at www.gavi.org)

WHO in 1974 formulated ***Expanded Programme of Immunization (EPI)*** for mass vaccination as a part of the public health program, and the program included vaccination against six diseases: tuberculosis (BCG), diphtheria, tetanus, pertussis (DTP vaccine), measles and poliomyelitis.

In the 1980s WHO expanded EPI with ***Universal Immunization Program (UIP)*** with the emphasis on expanding the vaccination coverage to every newborn child in the world. While EPI added more vaccines for immunization program, UIP aimed to expand coverage. The challenges were many and formidable: supply of quality vaccines, lack of reliable cold-chain and reach of healthcare delivery, awareness/education, funding, lack of enthusiasm on the part of local governments, and the ever-expanding list of vaccine-preventable diseases. Infant mortality has been reduced from 12.6 million in 1990 to 6.3 million in 2013 (Kang 2017, Madhavi 2005). While vaccination has proved its value in reducing infant mortality in many countries, it still remains high in other countries, primarily because of lack of full vaccination coverage (see Figure 1).

In the early phase, a full support from many underdeveloped countries was not forthcoming for a variety of reasons. Lately, though, most of the countries have realized the importance of vaccination program in development of their human resources and we are seeing encouraging results. Considering millions of deaths prevented by vaccination, EPI is considered to be one of the most successful public health programmes to date. In 1980, global immunization coverage for the first dose of the *Diphtheria-Tetanus-Pertussis (DTP)* vaccine was 30% and 20% for the third dose (DTP3). By 1990, global coverage for these two vaccinations had reached 88% and 76% respectively, and by 2012, it reached 91% and 83% (see Figure 2).

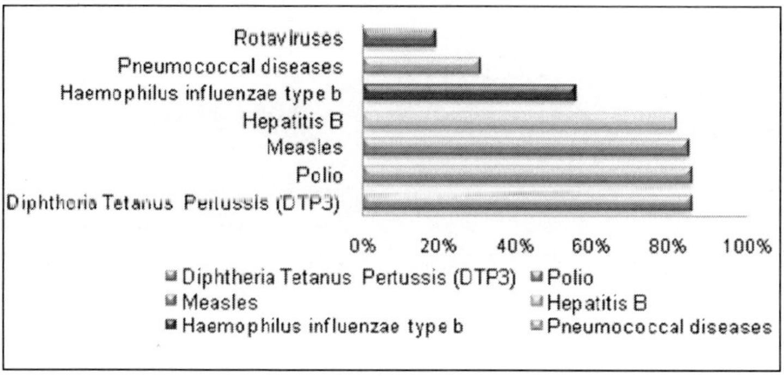

Fig. 2: Global Immunization Coverage for Six EPI Vaccines in 2014

1.2 History of Vaccines in India

History of vaccines in India is as old as the history of vaccine development in the world. During the latter half of the 19th century, fifteen vaccine institutes were established in India, primarily as a response to the death of many British in India due to tropical infections. The institutions' contribution was remarkable—development of the first vaccine for plague in 1897 and the vaccine for cholera in the same year, both in India. The institutes were also involved in the manufacturing of vaccines like TT, DT, DPT *etc.* Post-independence was an era of neglect and lull because many of these initial vaccine institutions became obsolete or irrelevant. It took India 30 years to develop the first policy document on vaccination (WHO 2015). Some of the earlier institutions like Hoffkine Institute, Central Research Institute in Kasauli, Pasteur Institute of India were revitalized and new government-backed public sector undertaking units were formed, primarily, to meet the demand for the vaccines for the expanded public vaccination program.

1.3 Vaccination Coverages

Since the start of the EPI in 1974, the proportion of the world's children who receive their basic vaccines has increased from 15 percent to nearly 90 percent. The goal now is to reach at least 90% of the population nationally, and at least 80% in every district. In 2012, 59 countries had already achieved this target including several low- and middle-income countries (GVR 2014, UIP 2010). For India complete immunization is still below 70% while individual coverage may be about 80–85% (UIP 2010). According to WHO and GAVI, 18 million children are undervaccinated in the world, and one-third of them reside in India (see Figure 3), followed by Nigeria, Pakistan, and Ethiopia (GAVI 2019,

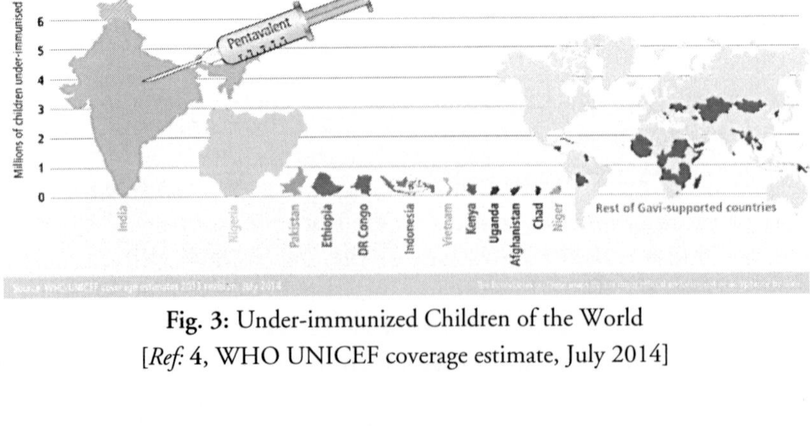

Fig. 3: Under-immunized Children of the World

[*Ref:* 4, WHO UNICEF coverage estimate, July 2014]

WHO 2015). Children from the sub-Saharan region and Southern Asia still face a higher risk of dying before their fifth birthday. There are still several countries where the infant mortality rate (death before 5 yrs age per 1000 live births) is 80 or more and the target remains of 25 or less. Most of the infant mortality is due to the diseases that can be prevented by proper vaccination. The number of unvaccinated children has fallen during the past decade in some but not all large countries. Nigeria, Pakistan, and Brazil are the examples of the countries where a number of unvaccinated children (for example, DTP3) have increased.

The current decade (2011-2020) is declared as the ***decade of vaccines*** by the WHO. To achieve full coverage, WHO designed and floated the GVAP with the commitment from member countries (UIP 2010, WHO 2012). The mission outlined in the GVAP is straightforward: improve health by extending the full benefits of immunization to all people, regardless of where they are born, who they are, or where they live (WHO 2012). An estimated one in five children still does not receive the basic EPI vaccines. GVAP plans to reach and vaccinate every child in each and every corner of the world. Ambitious it sounds but worth committing to reap the real benefits of vaccines in reducing the disease burden among young children. The vision for the Decade of Vaccines (2011–2020) is of a world in which all individuals and communities enjoy lives free of vaccine-preventable diseases.

2. CHALLENGES

2.1 Awareness and Education

Vaccination may be very good for the prevention and elimination of diseases from the population, however, its effects and therefore appreciation is not immediate. It takes decades of intense efforts to see its outcome(s). Moreover, some of the earlier vaccines and a few of the new vaccines have occasionally shown adverse effects in some individuals raising the doubt about both the diverse individualized response and the safety of vaccination. To add to this, there are advocacy groups and ancient beliefs working against the goal of full coverage. To counter this, a long-term sustained effort is required at every level. Developing countries have several other priorities and vaccination takes a back seat as its outcome is not instant. Once a political fraternity is roped into the vaccination campaign, the rest of the problems are easy to overcome.

2.2 Vaccine Production and Availability

The global market for vaccines has witnessed over 20% of annual growth during the past 15 years (NEA 2017) (see Figure 4). Although much of the growth is because of increased demand in the West, until now the vaccine production was confined to about a dozen major players both in the USA and Europe. Globally GSK, Pfizer, Merck, Sanofi Takeda and Diachi Sankyo are the major vaccine suppliers.

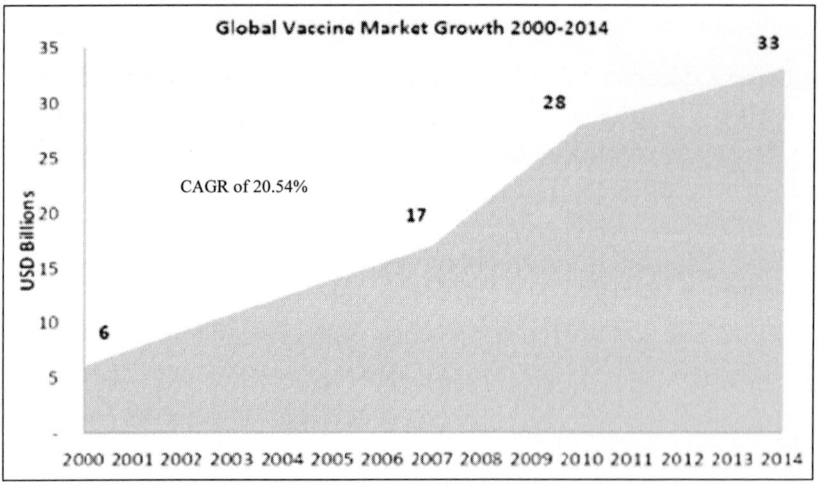

Fig. 4: The Growth of Vaccine Market in the World

The ambitious goal of reaching every child for vaccination is a laudable goal but do we have enough vaccines available and affordable in every village in each country? Under the circumstances even if the availability is assured, affordability is also a major barrier. There is negligible production in much of the developing world where vaccines were much needed in large numbers, and the high cost of these vaccines is a major barrier. To make vaccine products available as well as affordable, vaccines should be produced locally, if not in every country then in a regional production hub. With a few exceptions like India, China, Brazil, and South Africa, local production has not yet been realized (Figure 5). The Significant contribution to the production of vaccines in the developing countries is reflected in the procurement of vaccines by UNICEF from developing the world (UNICEF 2016, WHO 2016).

Since the 1980s, the quality of vaccines has been assured, through the prequalification system managed by the WHO, so that these vaccines can be recommended for bulk purchase by UNICEF, ***GAVI Alliance*** (formerly known as the Global Alliance for Vaccines and Immunization) and other funding agencies. Thanks to prequalification and other regulatory reforms, the vaccines used in national immunization programs are generally of an assured quality.

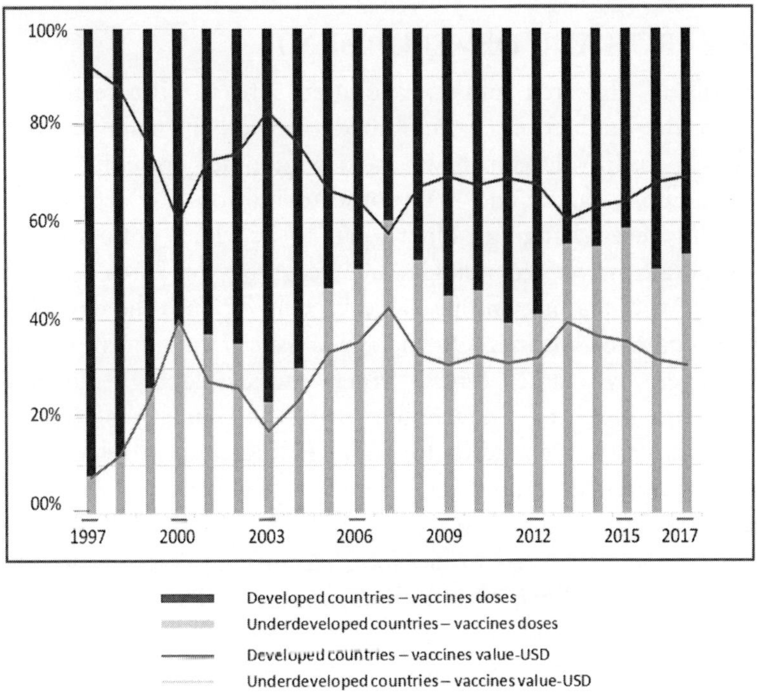

Fig. 5: UNICEF Procurement from Developing Countries 54% by volume, and 30% by Value of Vaccines Procured by UNICEF are from Developing Countries

2.3 Cold Chain and Distribution Infrastructure

Good vaccination coverage requires efficient transportation and distribution to the remotest areas of the country. There is a remarkable improvement in road and air transportation in many developing countries. However, vaccines require a cold-chain distribution network which is still missing in many countries. Better roads, cold-chain distribution along with good communication infrastructure in rural areas will certainly help to achieve the ambitious target of GVAP.

2.4 Funds and Affordability

As discussed earlier, governments in the developing economies look for low hanging fruits and fail to see the long-term potential of vaccination, and hence it results in low priority for the available scarce funding. High price for vaccines demanded by foreign multinational corporation (MNCs) limits the efforts of poorer countries. Better economic outlook in these countries and possible regional production can alleviate countries from such bottleneck and vaccination can become affordable.

3. RESEARCH AND DEVELOPMENT

The Goals of Research and Development are to (i) streamline and economize the production of established vaccines, (ii) make vaccine safe and efficacious, (iii) develop new vaccines for other preventable diseases like HIV, Ebola, cancer and many other conditions, (iv) cope up with newer and ever-changing older pathogens like influenza virus, (v) incorporate newer technologies like recombinant DNA technology, DNA based vaccination, epitope-based vaccine *etc.* into the development of new or improved vaccines. One unsettled issue is the concern that R&D is still driven by market forces. When the developing countries are grappling the issues of the manufacturing and supply of 'approved' affordable vaccines, their needs for more efficacious and relevant newer vaccines are ignored. Hopefully, ***Coalition for Epidemic Preparedness Innovations (CEPI)*** will be able to prioritize R&D needs of the developing world. There is also a need to develop thermo-stable vaccines which can withstand extreme climatic conditions *i.e.* disruptive power supply or vaccines that can be delivered child-friendly needle-free delivery methods. Padh and Desai (2018) have outlined development of orally deliverable *Shigella* vaccine candidates through *Lactobacilli* (Padh and Desai 2019, Unpublished data). The science of pharmaco-genetics dictates that genetically every individual is unique and any pharmaceutical or vaccine product cannot be equally effective in all of the major population groups, necessitating the need to consider genetics of the target population while developing a vaccine.

To add to the complexity of vaccine design, many pathogens have evolved mechanisms to change themselves (Rappuoli 2007). As shown in Figure 6, HIV changes its antigens almost every day while influenza virus changes itself every year and pneumonia and meningitis bacteria change every 10 years. Fortunately, few pathogens decided to cooperate and do not change much over a period of time and are easier target for vaccine design. At the beginning of the season, WHO predicts and declares the version of influenza strains predicted to appear during the coming winter season and the industry struggles to be ready with the appropriate and effective vaccine for the predicted strain. Strain variation adds complexity in vaccine design and makes the timely availability of effective vaccines a major challenge.

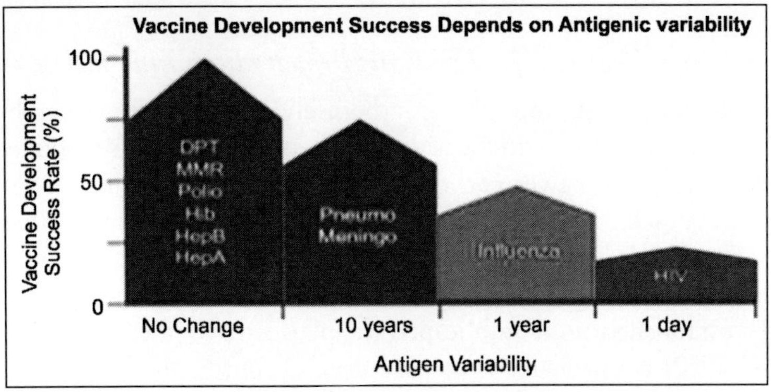

Fig. 6: Variations in Pathogens Requiring Frequent Newer Vaccines (Rappuoli, 2007)

3.1 Newer Technologies and New Generation Vaccines

We have come a long way since varioles were first used for vaccination. Subsequently, live or attenuated pathogens were used and then antigenic molecules were adopted for the vaccination purpose. With each step, vaccines became safer than the previous generation vaccines, and in some cases better efficacious. Advances in molecular biology provided better tools for designing better, safer or targeted vaccines. Computational science helped to see the antigen molecules in finer details and pick out portion(s) of the antigen molecule responsible for inducing protective immune response (Padh and Desai, 2018). Efforts are also underway to develop long-lasting vaccine preparations and vaccines which are amenable to easy delivery through oral or nasal route (Padh and Desai 2019, unpublished data). With time, we will see that vaccines used for public vaccination program will also reap the benefits of newer technologies for public good.

3.2 Avenues to Full Vaccination Coverage

The above points discussed two major areas: (**a**) How to ensure supply of current as well as future vaccines through intense R&D to ensure both their efficacy and safety, and (**b**) How to penetrate coverage to the remotest part of the world, particularly in the poor and developing countries. To coordinate activities in these two domains, WHO, UNICEF, the World Bank, and several other philanthropists have joined together and established the following two agencies: 1) ***Coalition for Epidemic Preparedness Innovation*** (***CEPI)*** to coordinate the newer and safer vaccine development initiatives mentioned above, and 2) ***The Global Alliance for Vaccines and Immunization (GAVI)*** for increasing the immunization coverage to the remote areas.

3.2.1 *CEPI—Coalition for Epidemic Preparedness Innovation*

Pathogens are smart and change themselves frequently enough that available vaccines prove ineffective as discussed earlier (see Figure 6). Moreover, there are newer pathogens and reemerging pathogens that are perhaps best tackled with the preventive vaccines. In addition, there are numerous infections for which vaccines are desirable but not available. To keep the world prepared for such potential epidemics, CEPI was recently established as a public-private platform to focus on R&D of vaccines. CEPI is a new alliance to finance and coordinate the development of new vaccines to prevent and contain infectious diseases and is funded by several governments, The World Economic Forum, The Bill and Melinda Gates Foundation, The Welcome Trust and others (CEPI 2019). For further information about CEPI and its activities, visit *www.cepi.net*

3.2.2 *GAVI—The Global Alliance for Vaccines and Immunization*

GAVI—the Vaccine Alliance, it was established in the year 2000. Immunization received a massive boost in 2000 with the launch of the GAVI Alliance (Figure 7), bringing together governments, international

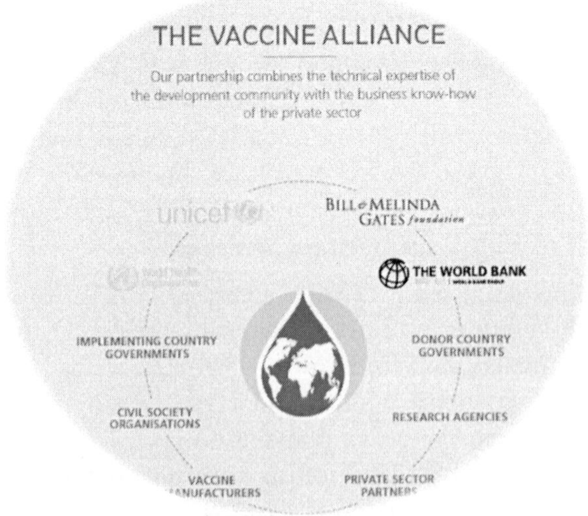

Fig. 7: GAVI, the Vaccine Alliance *[Ref. 1]*

agencies, the private sector and philanthropic foundations like BMGF, The Welcome Trust. GAVI Alliance has made a major contribution to improving access to sustainable immunization services in the partner countries (GAVI 2019). Still, many countries are falling short of the ambitious goals set out in the 2020 Global Vaccine Action Plan (**GVAP**) that countries adopted at the World Health Assembly in 2012.

4. INDIAN SCENARIO IN VACCINATION AND VACCINE PRODUCTION

India had a very good start in the area of vaccine development and vaccine production. As outlined earlier, India had set up several institutions in the nineteenth century which helped the development of vaccines for plague as well as cholera, and subsequently were utilized for vaccine production for the mass vaccination program. Post-independence, it took India 3 decades to wake up to the importance of vaccination as a public health issue. In 1978 Expanded Immunization Programme was adopted in India, which was introduced earlier in 1974 by the WHO. The programme gained momentum in 1985 and was expanded as the Universal Immunization Programme (UIP) to be implemented in a phased manner to cover all districts in the country by 1989–90 (UIP 2017). In India, Immunization has helped bringing down the annual mortality of children under five from 3.3 million to 1.3 million per year (Madhavi 2005). As shown in Figure 8, India demonstrated that since 1978 when it adopted the WHO's

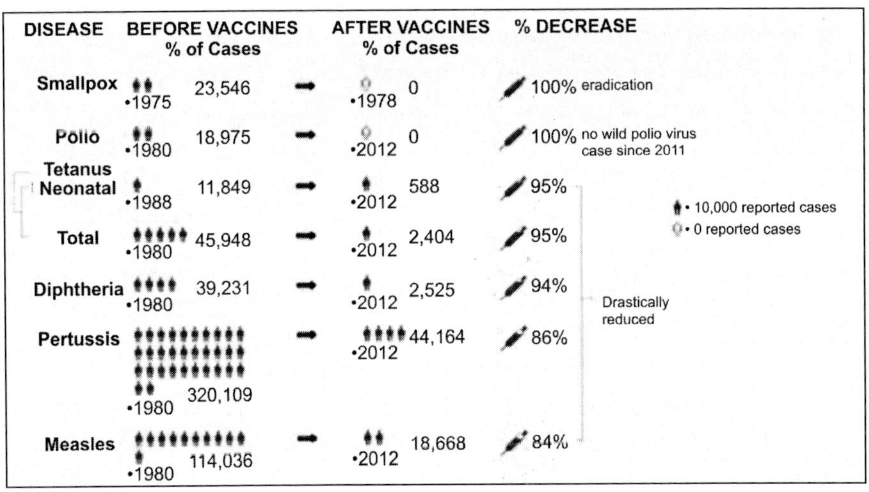

Fig. 8: India: Effective Vaccination Program

(*Source:* UNICEF India)

EPI vaccination program eradication of a number of diseases and reduction of the burden of the rest became a reality. Nevertheless, for a variety of reasons, coverage for vaccination is not as good as it can be, and India has the most under vaccinated children in the world and as a result, one-third of the world's infant mortality is in India. In India, the complete vaccination is still less than 70%. With Indian economy on a good trajectory for the past 15 years and with a number of quality vaccine manufacturers in India, it is time India has to come out of this dubious distinction of having the most under vaccinated children. As one newspaper recently reported, "*India leads in vaccine production but not in vaccination*". It is time for India to shake off this image and realize its vast population as a demographic dividend by saving lives and improving the quality of lives of its children.

5. VACCINE MANUFACTURING IN INDIA

Post-independence some of the vaccine institutions set up earlier by the British were used for the manufacturing of vaccines in India. Subsequently, India set up several of its own units for the manufacturing of vaccines as a Public Sector Undertaking (PSUs). Over the period of time, many of such PSUs proved to be of little value as they did not adopt newer technologies and could not cope up with the increased demand for public vaccination programs. Private players were then permitted to enter vaccine production as a part of liberalization. Now India has government-owned manufacturing units—*Central Research Institute in Kasauli, Pasteur Institute of India in Coonoor*; Public Sector Units—*Bharat Immunological and Biological Corporation Ltd.* and Private players like *Bharat Biotech International Ltd.*, and *Serum Institute of India Ltd.* While PSUs played major role during the post-independence era, currently the private players are dominant in vaccine manufacturing. As seen in Figure 9, vaccine procurement by UNICEF from India has grown with an annual growth rate of about 25% during the past 15 years (UNICEF 2016, WHO 2016). This has placed India firmly on the world map of vaccine production. UNICEF procures about 234 vaccine preparations of about 145 vaccines. Indian manufacturers provide 95 of these 234 preparations (UNICEF 2016, WHO 2016). One estimate is that every second child in the world is vaccinated with a vaccine manufactured in India. It is hoped that India's potential in vaccine manufacturing will translate into better vaccination coverage.

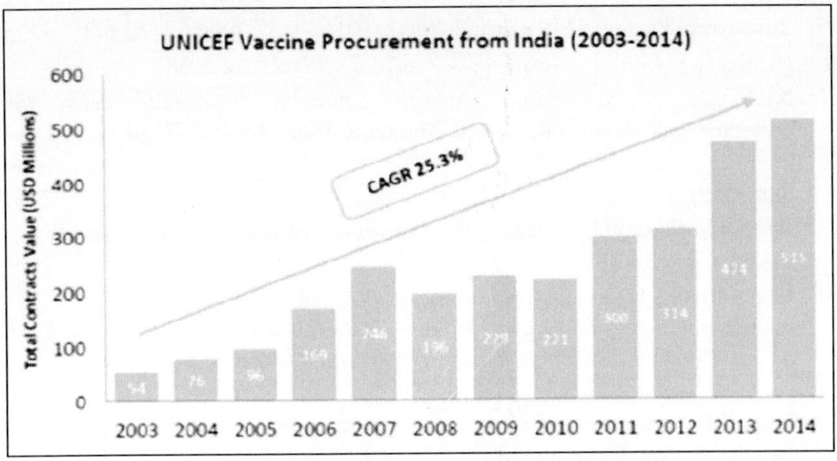

Fig. 9: UNICEF Procurement of Vaccines from India
(*Source:* UNICEF India)

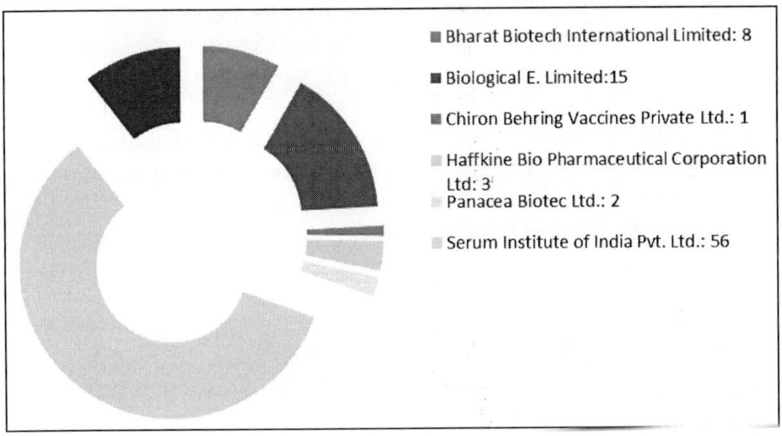

Fig. 10: UNICEF Procurement of Vaccines from Major Manufacturers in India
(*Source:* UNICEF India)

REFERENCES

[1] CEPI (2019). CEPI – Coalition for Epidemic Preparedness Innovation. www.cepi.net

[2] Gagandeep, Kang (2017). Vaccines and Public Health in India. https://www.ias.ac.in/MYM2017/public/pdf/14_GagandeepKang.pdf

[3] GAVI (2019). The Global Alliance for Vaccines and Immunization. The Vaccine Alliance, www.gavi.org

[4] GVR (2014). Grand View Research 2014. Market Research Report, Report ID: 978-1-68038-990-6. https://www.grandviewresearch.com/industry-analysis/vaccine-market

[5] https://mohfw.gov.in/sites/default/files/41016395871489662752.pdf

[6] Madhavi, Y. (2005). Vaccine policy in India. *PLoS Med* 2: 387–391.

[7] NEA (2017). Netherlands Enterprise Agency, 2017. Rijksdienst voor ondernemend. Report on Vaccine Market in India. www.RVO.nl

[8] Padh, H. and Desai, P. (2018). Subunit and epitope based vaccine for Shigellosis:

[9] Rappuoli, R. (2007). Bridging the knowledge gaps in vaccine design. *Nature Biotechnology* 25: 1361–66.

[10] UIP (2010). Universal Immunization Program – Reaching Every Child. Ministry of Health and Family Welfare, Government of India, 2010, p. 1–88. http://www.who.int/immunization/programmes_systems/financing/countries/cmyp/india_cmyp_2013-17.pdf

[11] UIP (2017). Universal Immunization Programme, Ministry of Health and Family Welfare, Government of India 2017.

[12] UNICEF (2016). UNICEF India. www.unicef.in

[13] UNICEF (2016). UNICEF Supply Division. https://www.unicef.org/supply

[14] Use of r-*Lactobacilli* for antigen delivery. Unpublished Data.

[15] WHO (2010). WHO Strategic Plan 2010-15, Department of Immunization, Vaccines and Biologicals 2010. p. 1–28. http://www.who.int/immunization/documents/IVB_SP_2010-15_final_Ver.pdf

[16] WHO (2012). World Health Organization, Global Action Vaccine Plan 2011–2020, p. 1–148 2012. http://www.who.int/immunization/global_vaccine_action_plan/GVAP_doc_2011_2020/en

[17] WHO (2015). WHO-UNICEF report on Vaccine Coverage Estimate 2015. http://apps.who.int/immunization_monitoring/globalsummary/timeseries/tswucoveragedtp3.html

[18] WHO (2016). Supply of vaccines. https://extranet.who.int/gavi/PQ_Web

Vaccination Strategies of the Blood-Borne Viruses in Africa: Current Status and Future Insight

Rola Nadeem* **and Mahmoud Mohamed Bahgat**

Department of Therapeutic Chemistry, Division of Pharmaceutical and Drug Industries, Research and Research Group Immune- and Bio-markers for Infection, the Centre of Excellence for Advanced Science, The National Research Centre, Dokki, Giza 12311, Egypt

E-mail: *rola.nadeem@hotmail.com

ABSTRACT: This chapter highlights the status of the available vaccination strategies against blood-borne viruses in Africa either as an in-action strategy as in Ebola virus, hepatitis B and E viruses or a clinical trial approaching approval as in human immunodeficiency virus and the on-going trials on hepatitis C virus vaccine development. This review presents a brief overview over epidemiology and the risk groups in Africa, as well as further insights stated in the future plans and the frameworks put within the achievement of the sustainable development goals. We stressed on the drastic impact and increased prevalence of such diseases in Africa that emphasizes the urgency of either developing specific vaccines or the evaluation of the current vaccine's efficacy for its studying its application in Africa.

Keywords: Blood-borne Viruses, Ebola Virus, HBV, HCV, HEV, HIV, Vaccine, Decade of Vaccine, Global Vaccination Action Plan.

1. INTRODUCTION

Africa is characterized by high incidence of both communicable and non-communicable diseases. The region is one of the major foci in the world-wide health improvement strategies towards improvement of public health infrastructure to ensure equity in treatment and protection of all inhabitants. The World Health Organization (WHO), African Regional Office adopted a transformation agenda (WHO 2017h) and developed health programs and strategies that reflect vision and targets of the United Nations health-related Sustainable Development Goals (SDGs). Such programs focus on solving the difficulty of the African health problems by enhancing the infrastructure, medical products, delivery systems, surveillance and coverage of information systems. Additionally, by improving health related services through increasing access to essential services, quality of services and the resilience of the system. Moreover, the importance of the health system performance development in accessing the risk factors and the possible efficient means of lowering the morbidity and mortality rates are paramount (WHO 2018e).

Among the common infectious communicable diseases in Africa are the blood-borne infections. Those are defined as the infections where the etiological agent circulates in blood stream and could be transmitted through direct contact between infected blood and contaminated body fluids with uninfected individual's blood through wounds or other invasive procedures (Pirozzolo *et al.,* 2007). Despite that most of the infectious diseases causes sepsis or viremia not all blood circulating infections can be defined as blood-borne, whereas the definition is restricted to the blood route of transmission. According to this restricted definition, blood-borne viruses (BBV) are delimited to human immunodeficiency virus (HIV), hepatitis viruses B and C (HBV and HCV, respectively) as the most commonly known blood-borne viruses. However, despite that the major route of transmission for the Hepatitis E virus (HEV) (Pischke *et al.,* 2016) and Ebola virus causing Ebola viral disease (EVD) (OSHA fact sheet, CDC, 2018a) is not the blood route, those two viruses are classified as less known facultative or not 'true' blood-borne viruses. The years prior to and following 2013 were, considered the peak of treatment strategies, where developed medicines and medical treatment cohorts focused on and showed success in lowering the morbidity and mortality rates of most of the communicable diseases. At a parallel occurrence, in May 2012, the World Health Assembly approved the framework of the Decade of Vaccines (DoV) (2011–2020) focusing on the importance of immunezation and vaccination. This framework was put forward within the Global Vaccine Action Plan (GVAP) with a clear mission as "to improve health by extending, by 2020 and beyond, the full benefits of immunization to all people, regardless of where they are born, who they are, or where they live" (WHO 2013a).

Success of immunization programs of developed or newly introduced vaccines, in combination with other health care and development interventions, lead to an effective decline in morbidity rates that exceeds in some extents the effectiveness of medical therapy or increases the effectiveness of treatments. This factual observation was obvious in reporting that focusing on vaccinating children under five years—along with improving health care and development interventions—resulted in falling down of annual number of deaths among children from an estimate of 9.6 million in 2000 to 7.6 million in 2010, despite the increase in number of children born each year (WHO 2013a). Vaccination not only contributes in lowering prevalence of some infections (as in case of hepatitis B virus and *Haemophilus influenzae* type b) but also in a nearing eradication of such disease (as in case of smallpox and poliomyelitis). The developed strategies worldwide and in particular those focusing on the African region are targeted towards the development of current vaccination strategies and research on vaccine discovery for globally recognized communicable diseases.

However, the available vaccinations do not cover all the infectious diseases known. The available licensed vaccines are used to prevent and control 25 known bacterial or viral infections (WHO 2013a, IFPMA 2015). This limited number of immunization-targeted infections are due to the efficient vaccine development of complex processes. This process starts with extensive basic laboratory research to identify immunogenic antigens or formulations to a series of pre-clinical studies for the efficiency and the safety of the vaccine candidate in *ex-vivo* and *in-vivo* systems that depend primarily on the availability of proper representative cell culture line and animal model as well as the success of the candidate to provoke immune response. This pre-clinical stage includes numerous adaptations and potential of vaccine candidates to pass to clinical trials stage. Clinical trials encompass the efficacy evaluation reports on the tolerance of the formulation, the target age group and the efficacy in special patient groups that responds to the vaccination trials (Parkman *et al.,* 1999). This long sensitive procedure made the vaccine registry and approval more limited than expected.

Reporting on countries or regions herein is based on according to the region classification used in the WHO reports. Using "Africa" or "African countries" as used in the text refers to the whole African continent including its islands whereas. Using "African region" refers to the WHO African region (AFR) definition that includes 47-member states in Africa excluding the Northern countries (Somalia, Djibouti, Sudan, Egypt, Libya, Tunisia, Morocco) where those seven (7) countries are among the WHO Eastern Mediterranean Region (EMR) (WHO, 2018e, WHO EMRO). Using "Sub-Saharan" region refers to the UNICEF classification of the African countries into: Middle East and North Africa, as well as Eastern, Southern, West and Central Sub-Saharan regions (UNICEF, 2017). The latter definitions apply unless the country is stated by name.

This chapter reports on the current status of the available vaccination strategies against BBVs (see Table 1) in Africa either as an in-action strategy or a clinical trial approaching approval. We stressed on the drastic impact and increased prevalence of such diseases in Africa that emphasizes the urgency of the vaccination approaches in the Region either by developing vaccines or the evaluation of the current vaccine's efficacy for or studying its application in Africa.

Table 1: Highlights on the Approved or Near-Approved Vaccinations against BBVs

Virus	*Vaccine*	*Vaccine Status*	*Target Group*	*Country of Origin*	*Efficacy in Studied Age Groups*	*Ref.*
HBV	Recombivax HB Recombivax HB pediatric	Monovalent vaccine	Adults and pediatric	USA	0–1 year: 100% 11–15 years: 98–99% 20–39 years: 95–98% >40 years: 91%	McAleer 1984, Merck Canada 2012
	Engerix-B Engerix-B pediatric	Monovalent vaccine	Adults and pediatric	Belgium	0–1 year: >90% 1–2 years: 98% Adults<40 years: 99.5% Adults >40 years: 95%	André *et al.*, 1988, André *et al.*, 1989, Zhu *et al.*, 2017a
	GeneVac-B	Monovalent vaccine	Adult and pediatric	India	<1 year: 100% 20–50 years: 99.5%	Vijayakumar *et al.*, 2004, Vijayakumar *et al.*, 2007
	Shanvac-B	Monovalent vaccine	Adult and pediatric	India	<1 year: 100% 20–50 years 98.4%	Vijayakumar *et al.*, 2004, Vijayakumar *et al.*, 2007
	Twinrix Adult Twinrix Junior	Combined vaccine	Adults and pediatric	England	<1 year: 98% 18–60 years: 97.9%	Ambrosch *et al.*, 1994, Thoelen *et al.*, 1999
	Pediarix	Combined Vaccine	Pediatric	USA	<1 year: 100%	Shinefield *et al.*, 1999

Virus	*Vaccine*	*Vaccine Status*	*Target Group*	*Country of Origin*	*Efficacy in Studied Age Groups*	*Ref.*
HEV	HECOLIN	Monovalen t vaccine	Adults	China	16–65 years: 93.3%	Zhu *et al.*, 2010b
EDV	rVSV-ZEBOV	Monovalen t vaccine	Adults	Canada	100%*	Henao-Restrepo *et al.*, 2017
HIV	ALVAC-HIV and AIDSVAX B/E vaccine regimen	Trial candidate	Adults	Thailand	18–30 years 31.2%	Rerks-Ngarm *et al.*, 2009
	ALVAC-HIV and a bivalent subtype C gp120 protein vaccine with MF59 adjuvant	Trial candidate	Adults	Thailand / USA	18–35 years: NA	de Montingny *et al.*, 2018

* EDV vaccine efficiency reported on short time-based studies and is still questionable (Metzger *et al.*, 2018).

2. EBOLA VIRUS

2.1 Disease and Transmission

Ebola virus is a member of the *Filoviridae* family. It causes ***Ebola Virus Disease (EVD)*** that is a severe acute viral illness characterized by the sudden onset of fever and fatigue followed by impairment in both Kidney and Liver functions and in some cases internal and external bleeding. The virus was primarily transmitted to human through a wild animal 'zoonotic' while human to human to human route then the transmission among humans occurred occurs through direct blood contact with an infected blood or bloody body fluid or a deceased body (WHO 2016a).

2.2 Epidemiology

The virus was first known in 1976 through two simultaneous outbreaks. The first was in Yambuku, Democratic Republic of Congo (at that time 'Zaire') with Case Fatality Rate (CFR) of 88%, and then the second was in Nzara, Sudan with CFR of 53%. There was a re-emergence in Sudan in 1979 where 32 cases were recorded with 22 deaths (Sanchez *et al.*, 2007). No cases were reported till 1994, whereas a re-emergence of the virus lead to a series of outbreaks in the Central African Region that ended around 1996 (Amblard *et al.*, 1997). The very next report of the disease was in one of the largest epidemics in Uganda with 425 cases and 224 deaths (CDC 2001). During the 2013 and 2016 the West African Ebola outbreak (EVD) accounted for 11300 deaths. The most recent reported outbreak in the African region was in North Kivu province, that was first reported in August 2018 with a recorded (as of 15 September 2018) total cases of 142 (111 confirmed and 31 probable) and 97 deaths (66 confirmed and 31 probable). The EVD appears to be an exclusive to the African region among human host with CFR ranging between 25–90% in the past outbreaks (WHO 2016a).

2.3 Vaccination Strategy

There are 12 vaccine candidates that has been undergone or undergoing clinical trials (WHO, 2017g) among those candidates the experimental vaccine called rVSV-ZEBOV, that was found to be highly protective against the virus in a trial conducted by the WHO and other international partners in Guinea in 2015 (WHO 2015b, WHO 2017g). This vaccine was studied in a clinical trial involving 11841 people, among the 5837 people who received the vaccine, no Ebola cases were recorded 10 days or more after vaccination (WHO 2016a). Another Ebola vaccine candidate, the recombinant adenovirus type-5 Ebola vaccine, was evaluated in a phase II clinical trial in Sierra Leone in 2015 which induced an immune response within 28 days post vaccination that declines over six months thereafter (Zhu *et al.*, 2017b).

2.4 Future Insight

In August 2018, WHO launched the first approved Ebola vaccination using the rVSV-ZEBOV vaccine in North Kivu province starting with 3220 doses after the onset of the latest outbreak (WHO, 2018a). This vaccination campaign is still ongoing and yet to be reported on vaccine efficacy. However, On the other side, the control and containment of EVD outbreaks was one of the highest concerns in the WHO transformation agenda for the negative effect of the transmission of the infection from health workers to individuals which that has a negative impact on other immunization plans in the region on the said suffering from the outbreak (WHO 2017h).

3. HBV

3.1 Disease and Transmission

HBV is a member of *Hepadnaviridae* family which infects liver, causing both acute and chronic hepatitis. HBV is primarily transmitted through direct exposure to infected blood or bloody body fluids, where most of secretions (saliva, tears *etc.*) are considered clean if not contaminated with infected blood. It is most commonly transmitted from mother to child at birth (WHO 2018b). Development of infection to the chronic stage depends on age of the infected person. It was found that, in African regions, 80–90% of infants become infected during the first year of life and 30–50% of children who receive infection before age of 6 years progress to chronicity. In adults, less than 5% of infected population develops chronic infection, whereas, 20–30% of chronically infected adults develop cirrhosis and liver cancer (WHO 2018b). This emphasized the importance of targeting infants or children at birth or at a very young age in order to encounter the morbidity rate of the infection.

3.2 Epidemiology

Epidemiology of HBV is through classifying regional areas according to the prevalence of HB surface antigen (HBsAg) among populations; where high-prevalent areas (> 8%) such as Asia Pacific and Sub-Saharan African regions which (Sub Saharan Africa) accounts for 87890 deaths annually (WHO 2017d). Intermediate-prevalent areas (2–7%) as seen in North Africa (prevalence was estimated as 4% in Egypt, 2.2% in Libya, 4–7% in Tunisia) and Middle East (Benani *et al.,* 2015). Parts of Eastern and Southern Europe, parts of Latin America and South Asia belong to this group. Low-prevalent areas (< 2%) include Morocco, Australia, Asia, Northern and Western Europe, Japan, North America and some countries in South America (MacLachlan *et al.,* 2015, WHO 2018b).

3.3 Vaccination Strategy

A safe and effective vaccine against HBV has been available since 1982 that was first released in West Germany in May 1986 then in the USA in July of the same year (Huzair *et al.,* 2017). Afterwards, the commercially available HBV vaccination formulations expanded worldwide either in a monovalent vaccine (as ENGERIX-B® and RECOMBIVAX HB®) or in a combined vaccine for adults as TWINRIX® which is a combination of inactivated hepatitis A virus and HBsAg, or a combined vaccine for infants and young children such as a) combined hepatitis B, diphtheria, tetanus, acellular pertussis (DTaP) and inactivated poliovirus (IPV) vaccine (PEDIARIX®) (CDC 2018b). The first dose is given at birth followed by 2 or 3 doses to complete the primary series (WHO 2018b). Level of anti-HB antibody in the range of >100 U/l to >10 U/l is considered protective but this level might decrease with time where antibody levels should be rechecked with the importance of a booster dose of vaccination after 10–20 years of the initial immunization (Jack *et al.,* 1999, Pfaender *et al.,* 2016). Worldwide, vaccination is 95% effective in preventing infection and chronicity development. On the other hand, vaccination has contributed to decline of infection incidence in children of age under 5 years from 4.7% in the pre-vaccination era to 1.3% in 2015 (WHO 2018b). It was reported that the birth-dose vaccine to neonates in the first 24 hours prevents mother to child transmission of HBV in 80–95% of cases (Lee *et al.,* 2006, Zou *et al.,* 2012).

3.4 Future Insight

Despite the effectiveness of the vaccination strategies to continuously alter the epidemiological classification, African countries or regions are still classified within the high to intermediate prevalent regions and considered to be a 'hotspot' with 6.1% (60 million cases) of the African region were reported to be infected with HBV as described in the WHO 2017 report on Hepatitis Virus Diseases (WHO 2017f). It was observed that in spite of the regional reported coverage with 3 doses of HepB vaccine (HepB3) vaccination increased from 5 in 2000 to 76% in 2015 (WHO 2013a), however, this coverage has plateaued at 70-75% since 2009 (WHO 2016c, Breakwell *et al.,* 2017). As commonly observed in some local areas, the delivery of the birth-dose can be a challenge in communities where a large proportion of births occur outside health facilities, as a result, coverage is reduced to around 38%. The GVAP reported that the HBV vaccination is considered underutilized particularly in the African region (WHO 2013a). Unfortunately, most people with chronic viral hepatitis are not aware of their status, though the 2017 World hepatitis day report showed that only 9% of HBV-infected people are not subjected to the statistical surveillance in vaccination reports (WHO 2017i) and that the focus on HBV surveillance and vaccination should be prioritised in the upcoming years.

In June 2016, the World Health Assembly adopted the first 'Global Health Sector Strategy on Viral Hepatitis, 2016–2020'. The strategy calls for:

1. An increase in routine childhood HBV vaccination coverage from 82% in 2015 to 90% by 2020, which will require strengthening of

overall childhood immunization programs along with specific efforts to target HBV vaccination for those people at increased risk (WHO 2016b)

2. Providing health workers with free immunization against vaccine-preventable diseases, including HBV vaccine
3. Providing HBV post-exposure prophylaxis vaccination as necessary (WHO 2016b) and
4. License of HBV vaccine in the ***Controlled Temperature Chain (CTC)*** in order to facilitate the vaccine delivery outside the cold chain to solve the coverage issue on births outside the health facilities (Petit *et al.,* 2017).

4. HCV

4.1 Disease and Transmission

HCV is a member of the *flaviviridae* family. The virus has seven (7) genotypes with more than 67 subtypes. It causes both acute and chronic hepatitis, where the acute infection is usually asymptomatic and about 15–45% of infected patients clear the infection within the first 6-months without any treatments. About 60–80% of infected patient develops chronic infection and of those about 15–30% is at of high risk to develop liver cirrhosis within 20 years (WHO 2018c). HCV is a blood-borne virus which can be transmitted through transfusion of infected blood or blood products and the reuse of infected needles or syringes among drug users or in poor hygiene healthcare units (WHO 2018c). Body fluids and secretions are considered clean unless contaminated with infected blood.

4.2 Epidemiology

Although hepatitis C is found worldwide with a prevalence in WHO regions varies from 0.5–1.0% (WHO 2018c), countries with high prevalence of HCV infection are located in eastern Europe, Asia, Sub-Saharan Africa and North Africa (Egypt with the highest HCV prevalence worldwide) (WHO 2017d). In HCV seroprevalence meta-analysis review in Africa (Riou J. *et al.*, 2015), it was reported that Egypt has the highest prevalence (14.7%) in North African region among adults, whereas other countries has much lower rate such as Algeria (2.0%) and Libya (1.2%). In West African region the highest prevalence is seen in Burkina Faso (6.1%), while other countries showed lower rates such as in as in Ghana (3.2%) and in Senegal (1%). In Central African region the highest prevalence is Cameroon (4.9%) others are Angola (3.9%), Rwanda (0.3%).

East African Regionhas a prevalent rate of 2.8% in Kenya to 1.3% in Mozambique while South African region showed lower rates from 1.6% in Namibia to 1.1% in South Africa (WHO, 2017a). The prominent HCV genotype (GT) varies among different African regions. In the Central Sub-Saharan region GT 4 is the most prominent with low frequencies of GT 1, 2 and 3. The Eastern Sub-Saharan Region has GT 4 and 2 are the most prominent with low frequencies of GT 3 and 5. In the Western Sub-Saharan area GT 1 and 2 are the most prominent with low frequencies of GT 4 while Southern Sub-Saharan Region had all genotypes reported except GT 6, with 5 as most dominant followed by GT 1 (Sonderup *et al.,* 2017). In North Africa and in particular Egypt the most prominent is GT 4 with lower frequencies of GT 1 and 3 (Karoney *et al.,* 2013).

4.3 Vaccination Strategies

There is no HCV vaccine currently available and the efficacy of the vaccine candidates subjected to trials mostly is restricted to one or two genotypes. Several prophylactic and therapeutic vaccine candidates reached the Phase-I and Phase-II clinical trials (Baumert *et al.,* 2014), however, at present no promising candidate has been approved for global or local use. Among prophylactic vaccine candidates used in clinical trials are:

4.3.1 *Core-ISCOMATRIX Vaccine*

Phase-I study using G1a core recombinant partial protein expressed in *Escherichia coli* system. It was found to be immunogenic and well tolerated, inducing more than 2-fold increase in T-cell cytokines in 7 of the 8 volunteers after 3 vaccination doses (Drane *et al.,* 2009).

4.3.2 *E1-E2-MF59C.1 Vaccine*

Phase-I study using GT-1a recombinant E1 and E2 glycoprotein expressed in Chinese Hamster Ovary cell line. The vaccine induced significant lympho-proliferative and antibody response and reported to be safe and well tolerated. However, there was no significant increase in the antibody response after the 3rd immunization suggesting an anamnestic response, beside that there was no significant difference in cytokine profile between immunized and placebo group (Frey *et al.,* 2010).

4.3.3 *Ad6NSmut and ChAd3NSmut Vaccines*

Phase-I study used multiple HCV non-structural (NS) proteins. Proteins were expressed using two adenoviral vectors based on two rare adenoviral serotypes human adenovirus 6 (Ad6) and Chimpanzee adenovirus 3 (ChAd3). The regimen showed acceptable tolerance and induced CD^4 and CD^8 T-cell response that were sustained for one year. The regimen induced neutralizing HCV-specific antibodies that were found to protect against both GT-1 and 3 (Branes *et al.,* 2012).

4.4 Future Insights

The HCV vaccine development process is still ongoing. In 2016 the World Health Assembly approved the health sector strategy on viral hepatitis as a contribution in the agenda of SDG by 2030. This strategy targets the elimination of hepatitis infection and in particular in hotspot countries like Egypt. The strategy depends primarily on direct acting anti-viral and the focus on health care-related malpractice improvement as a major cause of HCV transmission (WHO 2016b), where the vaccination development was completely absent from all plans.

5. HEV

5.1 Disease and Transmission

HEV is a member of the *Hepeviridae* family. The virus has at least 4 genotypes where GT-1 and 2 infect only human GT-3 and 4 occasionally infect human. In most cases it causes a self-limiting hepatitis that resolves in 2–6 weeks but it might lead to fulminate hepatitis (acute liver failure) that might lead to death (WHO 2017e). The primary route for HEV transmission is the fecal-oral route through contaminated water with the virus. However, it was also reported, in the international liver congress, that one-third of the chronic HEV cases are transmitted through blood products (Westhölter *et al.,* 2018). Although HEV is not a true blood-borne virus it is reported to be transmitted through blood transfusion and vertically from mothers to children (Pischke *et al.,* 2016, WHO 2017e).

5.2 Epidemiology

WHO estimates that HEV caused approximately 44000 deaths in 2015 (accounting for 3.3% of the mortality due to viral hepatitis), but the prevalence is highest in East and South Asia (WHO 2017e), Sub Saharan Africa and the Middle East (WHO 2013b). A country based systematic review which came out in the regional WHO report showed varying degree of HEV prevalence in the African region. In central African region, the sero-prevalence of HEV antibodies was 24% in Central African Republic, 0–14% in Gabon and 13% in Angola. In the East African region, HEV is responsible for 20–60% of overall acute hepatitis cases or among pregnant women. In the Southern African region, sero-prevalence varied from 5.8–19.1% and increased with age. In West African region, HEV was also responsible for 66% of acute sporadic hepatitis cases in Chad, at least 22% of such cases Cote d'Ivoire, 44% though; another study in Senegal failed to find any case. The reported sero-prevalence of anti-HEV antibodies in the region have varied from 4.4% in Ghana (increasing from 1% in school children to 8.1% in late adolescence), to 8% in Sierra Leone and 22% in Ghana (WHO 2010). In North Africa, the highest incidence was reported in both Egypt and Tunisia. In Egypt, the prevalence among chronic liver disease patients (23–62 years old) was reported as 80.1% (Abe *et al.,* 2006), while among blood donors (18–45 years old) was 45.3% (Abdel *et al.,* 1998). In a study on waste water treatment plants workers, it was found to be 50.6 to 51.2% (El-Esnawy *et al.,* 2000, Albatanomy *et al.,* 2011). In Tunisia, it was reported in poly-transfused patients as 28.7% (Hannachi *et al.,* 2011), while in random individuals of age above 60 to be 46% (Ben *et al.,* 1998).

Since 1979, more than 17 HEV outbreaks were recorded in the African region, with the most recent outbreaks taking place in Niger and Chad. It was reported as of May 2017, a total of 282 suspected cases including 27 deaths have been recorded. All reported deaths except for one were among pregnant women (mortality ratio: 9.6%) (WHO 2017c). Chad noted a total of 693 cases including 11 deaths of Acute Jaundice Syndrome (AJS) from September 2016 January 2017 (WHO 2017b). Another outbreak in South Sudan leading to 1203 HEV cases with 28 deaths was recorded from January 2013 to June 2014 (WHO 2014).

5.3 Vaccination Strategy

It was devastating to find that there is neither a specific treatment to HEV, where Ribavirin is described in case of chronic infection, nor a global vaccination available to face such high prevalence and frequent outbreak events (WHO 2017e). There are two available HEV vaccine candidates the first is a 56 kDa protein of HEV1 encoded in ORF2. It was found to be well tolerated with efficiency of 95% in phase II clinical trials. This vaccine is not registered or available for global use (Shrestha *et al.,* 2007). The second vaccine candidate is a 26 kDa protein of HEV1 encoded in ORF2 and known as HEV239 vaccine. It was found to be well tolerated with an efficacy of 98.7% in phase III clinical trials. This vaccine is registered and available in China and used in people aged >16 years old (Zhu *et al.,* 2010a) but not licensed outside of China.

5.4 Future Insight

The WHO did not recommend the routine use of the HEV293 vaccine in special patients' groups, pregnant women and children under 16 years due to the lack of sufficient studies on safety and efficacy of the vaccine in such groups (WHO 2015c). Efforts are currently underway to obtain WHO pre-qualification for emergency settings and in particular during the frequent HEV outbreaks occurring in the African regions (WHO 2017h, WHO 2018f). Despite the development of HEV293 HEV vaccine is still considered a vaccine under development (IFPMA 2015), it was completely absent from the future strategies of vaccine application in the DoV framework or the GVAP 2011–2020 plan.

6. HIV

6.1 Disease and Transmission

HIV is a member of the *Retroviridae* family. HIV targets immune cells causing CD^4 cell count depletion, leading to an overall immune deficiency in the patient. The most advanced stage of HIV infection is Acquired Immunodeficiency Syndrome (AIDS) that develops between 2 to 15 years from the onset of infection. The immune-deficiency caused by HIV/AIDS increases the susceptibility to infections (and in particular tuberculosis) and cancers, such infection are considered the major cause of deaths in HIV infection. In 2017, 940,000 people died from HIV-related causes globally (WHO, 2018d). HIV is a restricted blood-borne infection caused by the exchange of infected body fluids and infected blood transfusion. The major concern is the mother to child transmission either during pregnancy, labor or through infected breast milk, where the mother to child transmission rate is between 15–45% accounting for the high prevalence among children (WHO 2015a).

6.2 Epidemiology

The African Region accounts for two-third of the prevalence of HIV infection globally. There are 25.7 million individual living with HIV in the African region (WHO 2018d) with 2.3 million are children under the age of 15 years. Ninety percent (90%) of the children infected with HIV worldwide were reported in the Sub-Saharan African regions (WHO 2015a).

6.3 Vaccination Strategies

More than 200 HIV vaccine candidates have been clinically tested since 1986, of which only four reached the clinical trials (IAVI 2015). Globally, the first successful trial for the development of HIV vaccine was the RV144 Thai trial prior to 2009. The vaccine was a priming dose of recombinant canary pox vector vaccine (ALVAC-HIV) and two booster doses of recombinant glycoprotein 120 subunit vaccine (AIDSVAX B/E) vaccine regime. The ALVAC-HIV and AIDSVAX B/E vaccine regimen showed an efficacy of 60% in the first year and 31% after 3.5 years of follow up, however, the efficacy was statistically questionable but still considered a forward step toward a successful vaccine candidate (de Montingy *et al.,* 2018). This vaccine candidate priming dose is now used in a more advanced trials to improve its efficacy. The HIV Vaccine Trials Network (HVTN)—which is headquartered at the Fred Hutchinson Cancer Research Center, WA, USA—leads the HIV vaccine development through studies primarily funded by the National Institute of Allergy and Infectious Diseases (NIAID) of the National Institutes of Health (NIH), the network currently manages 18 active clinical trials of which three are large-scale in-human efficacy trials. Recently, announced the launch of one of the largest HIV vaccine trials in South Africa. The promising strong immune response reported during the HVTN 100 trial, which enrolled 252 HIV-negative adults lead to the initiation of the first advanced-phase large scale trial, under the code of HVTN 702 in South Africa. This phase 2b/3 randomized controlled trial (HVTN 702) started recruiting participants in October 2016, currently enrolling 5400 HIV negative adults of 18 to 35-year age range (NIH 2016, Abbasi 2017). This trial focus primarily on the development of the level and durability of the protection observed through the Thai trial vaccine. The HVTN 702 vaccine regimen consists of two experimental vaccines: a canarypox vector-based vaccine called ALVAC-HIV and a bivalent subtype C gp120 protein vaccine with MF59 adjuvant to enhance immune response (de Montingy *et al.,* 2018). There are no outcome reports available as the true start was in January, 2018.

6.4 Future Insight

The GVAP and the DoV plans besides focusing on the HIV vaccine development, are targeting and elimination of the HIV/AIDS disease through available antiretroviral drugs with a special focus on the elimination of mother to child transmission by 2020 (WHO 2013a). In January 2018, the WHO launched the *'Free to Shine'* campaign in the African region by the Organization of African First Ladies against

HIV/AIDS (OAFLA), the African Union and the WHO Regional Director for Africa. The campaign aims to accelerate actions to end childhood AIDS in the African Region by 2030 (WHO 2018f).

ACKNOWLEDGMENTS

The authors acknowledge the Egyptian Academy of Scientific Research and Technology for initiating the collaboration with the Centre for Science and Technology of the Non-Aligned and other Developing Countries and the National Research Center of Egypt for approving the collaboration and for providing all the logistics and facilities for preparing the chapter.

REFERENCES

[1] Abbasi, J. (2017). Large HIV vaccine trial launches in South Africa. *The Journal of the American Medical Association* 317: 350.

[2] Abdel, S.I., El-Din, M.S. and El-Din, M.E. (1998). A high hepatitis E virus (HEV) seroprevalence among unpaid blood donors and haemodialysis patients in Egypt. *The Journal of the Egyptian Public Health Association* 73: 165–179.

[3] Abe, K., Li, T.C., Ding, X., Win, K.M., Shrestha, P.K., Quang, V.X. *et al.* (2006). International collaborative survey on epidemiology of hepatitis E virus in 11 countries. *The Southeast Asian Journal of Tropical Medicine & Public Health* 37: 90–95.

[4] Albatanony, M.A. and El-Shafie, M.K. (2011). Work-related health effects among wastewater treatment plants workers. *International Journal of Occupational and Environmental Medicine* 2: 237–244.

[5] Amblard, J., Obiang, P., Edzang, S., *et al.* (1997). Identification of the Ebola virus in Gabon in 1994. *The Lancet* 349: 181–182.

[6] Ambrosch, F., Wiedermann, G., André, F. *et al.* (1994). Clinical and immunological investigation of a new combined hepatitis A and hepatitis B vaccine. *Journal of Medical Virology* 44: 452–456.

[7] André, F.E. and Safary, A. (1988). Clinical experience with a yeast-derived hepatitis B vaccine. In: Zuckerman AJ, ed. Viral Hepatitis and Liver Disease. Alan R Liss, Inc., New York, USA. Pp: 1025–1030.

[8] André, F.E. (1989). Summary of safety and efficacy data on a yeast-derived hepatitis B vaccine. *The American Journal of Medicine* 87: S14–S20.

[9] Barnes, E., Folgori, A., Capone, S., Swadling, L., Aston, S., Kurioka, A. *et al.* (2012). Novel adenovirus-based vaccines induce broad and sustained T-cell responses to HCV in man. *Science Translational Medicine* 4: 111–115.

[10] Baumert, T.F., Fauvelle, C., Diana, Y., Chen, D.Y. and Lauer, G.M. (2014). A prophylactic hepatitis C virus vaccine: A distant peak still worth climbing. *Journal of Hepatology* 61: S34–S44.

[11] Ben, M., Arrouji, Z., Slim, A., Lakhoua, R. and Ben Redjeb, S. (1998). Epidemiology of hepatitis E in Tunisia. *La Tunisie Medicale* 76: 129–131.

[12] Benani, A. (2015). Molecular epidemiology of HBV and HCV in North Africa In: 5Th World Congress on Virology. *Journal of Antivirals and Antiretrovirals* 7: 4.

[13] Breakwell, L., Tevi-Benissan, C., Childs, L., Mihigo, R. and Tohme, R. (2017). The status of hepatitis B control in the African region. *The Pan African Medical Journal* 27: 17.

[14] CDC (2001). Outbreak of Ebola hemorrhagic fever Uganda, August 2000–January 2001. Morbidity and mortality weekly report. Available online at: https://www.cdc.gov/mmwr/PDF/wk/mm5005.pdf. (Accessed Sep. 2018).

[15] CDC (2018a). Report on Ebola virus disease. Available at: https://www.cdc.gov/vhf/ebola/transmission/index.html (Accessed Sept. 2018).

[16] CDC (2018b). Report on Hepatitis B information. Available online at: https://www.cdc.gov/hepatitis/hbv/hbvfaq.htm (Accessed Sept. 2018).

[17] de Montigny, S., Adamson, B.J.S., Mâsse, B.R., Garrison, L.P. Jr., Kublin, J.G., Gilbert, P.B. and Dimitrov, D.T. (2018). Projected effectiveness and added value of HIV vaccination campaigns in South Africa: A modeling study. *Scientific Reports* 8: 6066.

[18] Drane, D., Maraskovsky, E., Gibson, R., Mitchell, S., Barnden, M., Moskwa, A. *et al.,* (2009). Priming of CD^{4+} and CD^{8+} T cell responses using a HCV core ISCOMATRIX vaccine: a phase I study in healthy volunteers. *Human Vaccines* 5: 151–157.

[19] El-Esnawy, N.A. and Al-Herrawy, A.Z. (2000). Seroprevalence of certain hepatitis viruses among Egyptian workers infected with Schistosomiasis. *The Journal of the Egyptian Public Health Association* 75: 357–366.

[20] Frey, S.E., Houghton, M., Coates, S., Abrignani, S., Chien, D., Rosa, D., *et al.* (2010). Safety and immunogenicity of HCV E1E2 vaccine adjuvanted with MF59 administered to healthy adults. *Vaccine* 28: 6367–6373.

[21] Hannachi, N., Boughammoura, L., Marzouk, M., Tfifha, M., Khlif, A., Soussi, S., Skouri, H. and Boukadida, J. (2011). Viral infection risk in polytransfused adults: seroprevalence of seven viruses in central Tunisia. *Bulletin de la Societe de Pathologie Exotique* 104: 220–225.

[22] Henao-Restrepo, A.M., Camacho, A., Longini, I.M. *et al.* (2017). Efficacy and effectiveness of an rVSV-vectored vaccine in preventing Ebola virus disease: final results from the Guinea ring vaccination, open-label, cluster-randomised trial (Ebola Ça Suffit!). *The Lancet* 389: 505–518.

[23] Huzair, F. and Sturdy, S. (2017). Biotechnology and the transformation of vaccine innovation: The case of the hepatitis B vaccine 1968–2000. *Studies in History and Philosophy of Biological and Biomedical Sciences* 64: 11–21.

[24] HVTN (HIV Vaccine Trials Network) website, (2018). Moving toward a much needed effective HIV vaccine. http://www.hvtn.org/en/media-room/news-releases/moving-toward-much-needed-effective-vaccine.html (accessed Sept. 2018).

[25] IAVI (2015). International AIDS Vaccine Initiative. Clinical Trials Database. Available online at: www.iavi.org (accessed Sept. 2018).

[26] IFPMA (2015). International Federation of Pharmaceutical Manufacturers and Associations. Delivering the promise of the Decade of Vaccines. Available online at: https://www.ifpma.org/wp-content/uploads/2016/01/IFPMA_Delivering_the_Promise_of_the_DoV_NewLogo.pdf(accessed Sep. 2018).

[27] Jack A.D., Hall A.J., Maine N., Mendy M., Whittle H.C. (1999). What level of hepatitis B antibody is protective? *Journal of Infectious Diseases* 179: 489–492

[28] Karoney, M.J. and Siika, A.M. (2013). Hepatitis C virus (HCV) infection in Africa: a review. *The Pan African Medical Journal* 14: 44.

[29] Lee, C., Gong, Y., Brok, J., Boxall, E.H. and Gluud, C. (2006). Effect of hepatitis B immunization in newborn infants of mothers positive for hepatitis B surface antigen: systematic review and meta-analysis. *The British Medical Journal* 332: 328–336.

[30] MacLachlan, J.H. and Cowie, B.C. (2015). Hepatitis B virus epidemiology. *Cold Spring Harbor Perspectives in Medicine* 5: a021410.

[31] McAleer, W.J., Buynak, E.B., Maigetter, R.Z., Wampler, D.E., Miller, W.J. and Hilleman, M.R. (1984). Human hepatitis B vaccine from recombinant yeast. *Nature* 307: 178–180.

[32] Merck Canada (2012). RECOMBIVAX HB Product monograph. Available online at: https://pdf.hres.ca/dpd_pm/00016542.PDF (Accessed Sept. 2018).

[33] Metzger, W.G. and Vivas-Martínez, S. (2018). Questionable efficacy of the rVSV-ZEBOV Ebola vaccine. *The Lancet* 391: 1021.

[34] NIH NIAID (2016). First new HIV vaccine efficacy study in seven years has begun. https://www.niaid.nih.gov/news-events/first-new-hiv-vaccine-efficacy-study-seven-years-has-begun (Accessed Sept. 2018).

[35] OSHA (2018). Occupational Safety and Health Administration. Fact sheet: Cleaning and decontamination of Ebola on surfaces. Washington, DC, USA. Available online at: https://www.osha.gov/SLTC/ebola/control_prevention.html (Accessed Sept. 2018).

[36] Parkman, P.D. and Hardegree, M.C. (1999). Regulation and testing of vaccines. In Plotkin SA, Orenstein WA, [eds.]. Vaccines, 3d ed. Philadelphia: Saunders.

[37] Petit, D., Tevi-Benissan, C., Woodring, J., Hennessey, K. and Kahn, A.l. (2017). Countries' interest in a hepatitis B vaccine licensed for the controlled temperature chain; survey results from African and Western Pacific regions. *Vaccine* 14: 6866–6871.

[38] Pfaender, S., Hahn, T., Steinmann, J., Ciesek, S. and Steinmann, E. (2016). Prevention strategies for blood-borne viruses in the era of vaccines, direct acting antivirals and antiretroviral therapy. *Reviews in Medical Virology* 26: 330–339.

[39] Pirozzolo, J.J. and LeMay, D.C. (2007). Blood-Borne Infections. *Clinics in Sports Medicine* 26: 425–431.

[40] Pischke, S., Hiller, J., Lütgehetmann, M., Polywka, S., Rybczynski, M., Ayuk, F. and Lohse, A. (2016). Blood-borne Hepatitis E Virus Transmission: A Relevant Risk for Immunosuppressed Patients. *Clinical Infectious Diseases* 63: 569–570.

[41] Rerks-Ngarm, S., Pitisuttithum, P., Nitayaphan, S., Kaewkungwal, J., Chiu, J., Paris, R., Premsri, N., Namwat, C., de Souza, M., Adams, E., Benenson, M., Gurunathan, S., Tartaglia, J., McNeil, J.G., Francis, D.P., Stablein, D., Birx, D.L., Chunsuttiwat, S., Khamboonruang, C., Thongcharoen, P., Robb, M.L., Michael, N.L., Kunasol, P., Kim, J.H. and Moph-Taveg, I. (2009). Vaccination with ALVAC and AIDSVAX to prevent HIV-1 infection in Thailand. *The New England Journal of Medicine* 361: 2209–2220.

[42] Riou, J., Aït, A.M., Blake, A., Vozlinsky, S., Brichler, S., Eholié, S., Boëlle, P.Y. and Fontanet, A. (2015). HCV epidemiology in Africa group. Hepatitis C virus seroprevalence in adults in Africa: a systematic review and meta-analysis. *Journal of Viral Hepatitis* 23: 244–255.

[43] Sanchez, A., Geisbert, T.W. and Feldmann, H. (2007). Filoviridae: Marburg and Ebola virus. In: Fields Virology, 5th Edition. Lippincott Williams & Wilkins, PHL, USA.

[44] Shinefield, H.R., Black, S., Ray, P., Chang, I.H., Lewis, N., Fireman, B. *et al.*, (1999). Safety and immunogenicity of heptavalent pneumococcal CRM197 conjugate vaccine in infants and toddlers. *Pediatric Infectious Diseases Journal* 18: 757–763.

[45] Shrestha, M.P., Scott, R.M., Joshi, D.M. *et al.* (2007). Safety and efficacy of a recombinant hepatitis E vaccine. *The New England Journal of Medicine* 356: 895–903.

[46] Sonderup, M.W., Afihene, M., Ally, R. *et al.* (2017). Hepatitis C in sub-Saharan Africa: the current status and recommendations for achieving elimination by 2030. *Lancet Gastroenterol Hepatol* 2: 910–919.

[47] Thoelen, S., Van Damme, P., Leentvaar-Kuypers, A., Leroux-Roels, G., Bruguera, M., Frei, P.C., Bakasenas, V. and Safary, A. (1999). The first combined vaccine against hepatitis A and B: An overview. *Vaccine* 17: 1657–1662.

[48] UNICEF (2017). Regional classification. Available online at: https://data.unicef.org/regionalclassifications. (Accessed Sept. 2018).

[49] Vijayakumar, V., Hari, R., Parthiban, R., Mehta, J. and Thyagarajan, S.P. (2004). Evaluation of immunogenicity and safety of Genevac B: A new recombinant hepatitis b vaccine in comparison with Engerix B and Shanvac B in healthy adults. *Indian Journal of Medical Microbiology* 22: 34–38.

[50] Vijayakumar, V., Subhadra, N., Saravanan, S., Suresh, S.J., Prasad, S.K. and Sadras, P.T. (2007). Comparison of three different recombinant hepatitis B vaccines: GeneVac-B, Engerix B and Shanvac B in high risk infants born to HBsAg positive mothers in India. *World Journal of Gastroenterology* 13: 3084–3089.

[51] Westhölter, D. *et al.* (2018). Presented at: International Liver Congress; Paris, France. Available online at: https://ilc-congress.eu/wp-content/uploads/2018/04/ILC-2018-Press-Kit_v3.pdf (Accessed Sept. 2018).

[52] WHO (2010). Report on The global prevalence of Hepatitis E virus infection and susceptibility: a systematic review. Available online at: http://apps.who.

int/iris/bitstream/handle/10665/70513/WHO_IVB_10.14_eng.pdf?sequence =1 (Accessed Sept. 2018).

[53] WHO (2013a). Report on Global Vaccine Action Plan 2011–2020. Available online at: http://www.who.int/immunization/global_vaccine_action_plan/GVAP_doc_2011_2020/en/ (Accessed Sept. 2018).

[54] WHO (2013b). Report on Plan of action for the prevention, care & treatment of viral hepatitis, Egypt 2014–2018. Available online at: http://www.emro.who.int/images/stories/egypt/VH_Plan_of_Action_FINAL_PRINT1.pdf (Accessed Sept. 2018).

[55] WHO (2014). Report on South Sudan: Family encourages early diagnosis and treatment after successful recovery. Available online at: https://www.afro.who.int/news/south-sudan-family-encourages-early-diagnosis-and-treatment-hepatitis-after-successful (Accessed Sept. 2018).

[56] WHO (2015a). Report on AFRO HIV/AIDS fact sheet. Available online at: https://afro.who.int/health-topics/hivaids (Accessed Sept. 2018).

[57] WHO (2015b). Report on first Ebola vaccine to be tested in affected communities one year into outbreak ring vaccination starts in Coyah, Guinea. Available online at: https://www.afro.who.int/news/first-ebola-vaccine-be-tested-affected-communities-one-year-outbreak-ring-vaccination-starts (Accessed Sept. 2018).

[58] WHO (2015c). Report on Hepatitis E vaccine: WHO position paper, May 2015. Available online at: http://www.who.int/wer/2015/wer9018.pdf?ua=1 (Accessed Sept. 2018).

[59] WHO (2016a). Ebola virus disease. Available online at: https://www.afro.who.int/health-topics/ebola-virus-disease (Accessed Sept. 2018).

[60] WHO (2016b). Report on Global health sector strategy on viral hepatitis 2016–2021: towards ending viral hepatitis. Available online at: http://apps.who.int/iris/bitstream/handle/10665/246177/WHO-HIV-2016.06-eng.pdf?sequence=1 (Accessed Sept. 2018).

[61] WHO (2016c). Report on Hepatitis B (HepB3) immunization coverage estimates by WHO region. Available online at: http://apps.who.int/gho/data/view.main.80300?lang=en (Accessed Sept. 2018).

[62] WHO (2017a). Nigeria employs numerous strategies to create awareness on viral hepatitis nationwide. Available online at: https://afro.who.int/news/nigeria-employs-numerous-strategies-create-awareness-viral-hepatitis-nationwide (Accessed Sept. 2018).

[63] WHO (2017b). Report on Disease outbreak – Hepatitis E- Chad- 24 January 2017 available online at: https://www.afro.who.int/health-topics/hepatitis/outbreak/24-january-2017-chad (Accessed Sept. 2018).

[64] WHO (2017c). Report on Disease Outbreak—Hepatitis E-Niger-5 May 2017. Available online at: https://www.afro.who.int/health-topics/hepatitis/outbreak/5-may-2017-niger (Accessed Sept. 2018).

[65] WHO (2017d). Report on Global hepatitis report, 2017. Available online at: www.who.int/hepatitis/publications/global-hepatitis-report2017/en/ (Accessed Sept. 2018).

[66] WHO (2017e). Report on Hepatitis E fact sheet. Available online at: http://www.who.int/en/news-room/fact-sheets/detail/hepatitis-e (Accessed Sept. 2018).

[67] WHO (2017f). Report on New hepatitis data highlight needs urgent global response. Available at: http://apps.who.int/iris/bitstream/handle/10665/255016/9789241565455-eng.pdf?sequence=1 (Accessed Sept. 2018).

[68] WHO (2017g). Report on Sage Ebola vaccination. Available online at: http://www.who.int/csr/resources/publications/ebola/sage-ebola-vaccination.pdf?ua=1(Accessed Sept. 2018).

[69] WHO (2017h). Report on The transformation agenda of the World Health Organization secretariat in the African region: phase 2; putting people at the center of change. Available online at: https://afro.who.int/sites/default/files/2018-05/Transformation%20Agenda%20Phase%202%20-%20Putting%20people%20at%20the%20center%20of%20change.pdf (Accessed Sept. 2018).

[70] WHO (2017i). Report on World Hepatitis Day 2017: Eliminate hepatitis. Available online at: http://www.who.int/campaigns/hepatitis-day/2017/event/en (Accessed Sept. 2018).

[71] WHO (2018a). Ebola vaccination begins in North Kivu. Available online at: http://www.who.int/news-room/detail/08-08-2018-ebola-vaccination-begins-in-north-kivu (Accessed Sept. 2018).

[72] WHO (2018b). Report on Hepatitis B Fact Sheet. Available at: http://www.who.int/en/news-room/fact-sheets/detail/hepatitis-b (Accessed Sept. 2018).

[73] WHO (2018c). Report on Hepatitis C fact sheet. Available online at: http://www.who.int/news-room/fact-sheets/detail/hepatitis-c (Accessed Sept. 2018).

[74] WHO (2018d). Report on HIV/AIDS fact sheet. Available online at: http://www.who.int/news-room/fact-sheets/detail/hiv-aids (Accessed Sept. 2018).

[75] WHO (2018e). Report on the state of health in the WHO African region: An analysis of the status of health services and health systems in the context of the Sustainable Development Goals. Available online at: https://afro.who.int/sites/default/files/2018-08/State%20of%20health%20in%20the%20African%20Region.pdf (Accessed Sept. 2018).

[76] WHO (2018f). Report on The work of the WHO in the African region: report of the regional director. Available online at: http://apps.who.int/iris/bitstream/handle/10665/273743/AFR-RC68-2-eng.pdf (Accessed Sept. 2018).

[77] WHO EMRO. Eastern mediterranean website. Available online at: http://www.emro.who.int/countries.html. (Accessed Sept. 2018).

[78] Zhu, F.C., Deckx, H., Roten, R., Michiels, B. and Sarnecki, M. (2017a). Comparative efficacy, safety and immunogenicity of Hepavax-Gene TF and Engerix-B recombinant hepatitis B Vaccines in Neonates in China. *The Pediatric Infectious Diseases Journal* 36: 94–101.

[79] Zhu, F.C., Wurie, A.H., Liang, Q. *et al.* (2017b). Safety and immunogenicity of a recombinant adenovirus type-5 vector-based Ebola vaccine in healthy adults in Sierra Leone: A single-centre, randomized, double-blind, placebo-controlled, phase 2 trial. *The Lancet* 389: 621–28.

[80] Zhu, F.C., Zhang, J., Zhang, X.F., *et al.* (2010a). Efficacy and safety of a recombinant hepatitis E vaccine in healthy adults: a large-scale, randomized, double-blind placebo-controlled, Phase-3 trial. *The Lancet* 376: 895–902.

[81] Zhu, F.C., Zhang, J., Zhang, X.F., Zhou, C., Wang, Z.Z., Huang, S.J., Wang, H., Yang, C.L., Jiang, H.M., Cai, J.P., Wang, Y.J., Ai, X., Hu, Y.M., Tang, Q., Yao, X., Yan, Q., Xian, Y.L., Wu, T., Li, Y.M., Miao, J., Ng, M.H., Shih, J.W. and Xia, N.S. (2010b). Efficacy and safety of a recombinant hepatitis E vaccine in healthy adults: a large-scale, randomized, double-blind placebo-controlled, Phase-3 trial. *The Lancet* 376: 895–902.

[82] Zou, H., Chen, Y., Duan, Z., Zhang, H. and Pan, C. (2012). Virologic factors associated with failure to passive-active immune prophylaxis in infants born to HBsAg-positive mothers. *Journal of Viral Hepatology* 19: e18–e25.

Mumps Outbreak among the School Students of Hebron District in Palestine, May 2015

Diaa O.H. Hjaija
Department of Preventive Medicine,
Palestinian Ministry of Health, Ramallah, Palestine
E-mail: pmdmoh@yahoo.com

ABSTRACT: In May, 20, 2015, Bait Kahel village-Hebron governorate primary health care clinic reported to the Central Preventive Medicine Department that 30 students in the village school were referred to the clinic with parotitis and fever within a one week period compared with zero reports of mumps case since February to the May, 20, 2015. A line listing of 761 cases was performed on a spreadsheet to ensure complete case investigation, and identification of affected population in Bait Kahel-Hebron governorate. The main affected age group was 9–14 years (669 cases). Analysis of the immunization status revealed that about 60.44% percent of affected population were vaccinated with a single dose of MMR, 12.22% received 2 doses of MMR, and about 27.34% whose immunization status was not known. More analysis of the situation was performed to identify the 30% of unknown immunization status showed that age group between 10–17 years only received one dose in routine EPI and was not targeted in any National Immunization Days (NIDs) or campaigns.

Keywords: Palestine, Outbreak, Hebron, Mumps, Vaccine, Preventable.

1. INTRODUCTION

Mumps is a vaccine preventable viral infection characterized by fever and inflammation of the salivary glands and whose complications include orchitis, deafness, and meningoencephalitis. In Palestine a recent cross sectional study including all notified cases of mumps in Gaza strip Palestine during the year 2013, a total of 1981 clinically diagnosed mumps cases were reported with an overall incidence of 116/100000. The majority of the cases 1181 (62.5%) were amongst males, age varied from one year to 83 years with a mean age of 13.7 years. Children of aged group 6 to 15 years who received only one dose of mumps vaccine have nearly

90.3% (1708) of cases, while 3.7% of cases received 2 doses and 6% of cases received no vaccine (Ghuneim and Dheir 2015). Another mumps outbreak in the West Bank lasted from December 2003 to June 2005, which occurred in Palestinian refugee camps of the West Bank. Sixty eight point one percent (2636/3871) of the cases were vaccinated with single dose of MMR vaccine, and the outbreak rates by camp ranged from less than 1 to 43 per 1000 population (overall 11/1000) as reported previously (Hindiyeh *et al.*, 2009). Thus, to promote the mass vaccination of MMR, a campaign was launched during May 2005.

Palestine is classified as an area with low mumps endemicity. The national incidence rate per 100,000 population was 2.2, 3.9, and 4.17 in 2012, 2011, 2010 respectively. In 2013 and 2014 the incidence rate per 100,000 increased to 46 and 432 respectively due to a mumps outbreak in Gaza strip. In Hebron Governorate where the current outbreak took place, the incidence rates per 100,000 population were 0.00, 0.00, 8.78 in 2013, 2014 and 2015 respectively (MOH 2016).

2. METHODOLOGY

The present study is a retrospective cohort study, which is a cohort of individuals that share a common exposure factor (immunization in this case) is compared with another group of equivalent individuals not exposed to that factor, to determine the factor's influence on the incidence of a condition (Mumps outbreak in this case). Vaccination status review of all cases birth between 1961–2014 were performed using SPSS ver. 20, all cases included in the current study were without any exclusion criteria.

3. RESULTS AND DISCUSSIONS

In May 20, 2015, Bait Kahel village of Hebron Governorate primary health care clinic reported to the Central Preventive Medicine Department that 30 students in the village school were referred to the clinic with parotitis and fever for a one week period compared with zero reports of mumps case since February to the May, 20, 2015.

Investigations of cases included: developing a case definition, case finding, interviews with primary cases, review of medical records and vaccination booklet were conducted. Cases were identified as residents of Hebron Governorate and classified according to the Preventive Medicine Department Policy Booklet that adopts the WHO clinical case definition, exposed contacts in schools and home were identified and control measures were immediately implemented through increase awareness of affected population. During the current outbreak a serosurvey was conducted by the Ministry of Health (MOH) on a sample of 113 school children selected from Hebron Governorate schools to determine their mumps immunoglobulin G (IgG) status. The result showed that 59.3% were positive for IgG, 34.5% were negative for IgG, and 6.2% Equivocal.

Table 1: Distribution of Mumps Cases by Age Group

No. of Cases	*Population Affected (in %)*	*Age Group Range*
53	7.0	0–4
132	17.3	5–8
440	57.8	9–14
80	10.5	15–19
19	2.5	20–24
14	1.8	25–29
11	1.4	30–34
5	0.7	35–39
3	0.4	40–44
2	0.3	45–49
2	0.3	50–54
761	**100.0**	**Total**

A line listing of 761 cases was performed on a spreadsheet to ensure complete case investigation, and identification of affected population in Bait Kahel - Hebron Governorate (see Table 1). The main affected age group was 9–14 years (440 cases) (Figure 1). Analysis of the immunization status revealed that about 60.44% percent of affected population was vaccinated with a single dose of MMR, 12.22% received 2 doses of MMR, and about 27.34% whose immunization status was not known (see Table 2 and Figure 2).

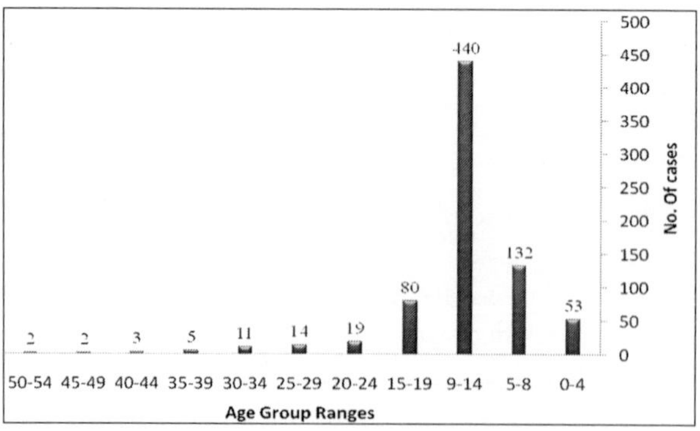

Fig. 1: Distribution of Mumps Cases by Age Group, Indicating the Highest Prevalence in 9–14 Years Age Group

More analysis of the situation was performed to identify the 30% of unknown immunization status showed that age group between 10–17 years only received one dose in routine EPI and was not targeted in any ***National Immunization Days (NIDs)*** campaigns.

Table 2: Immunization Status of Affected Population based on Doses

No. of Doses	*No. of Cases*	*Population Affected (%)*
One dose	460	60.45
two dose	93	12.22
Unknown	208	27.33
Total	**761**	**100**

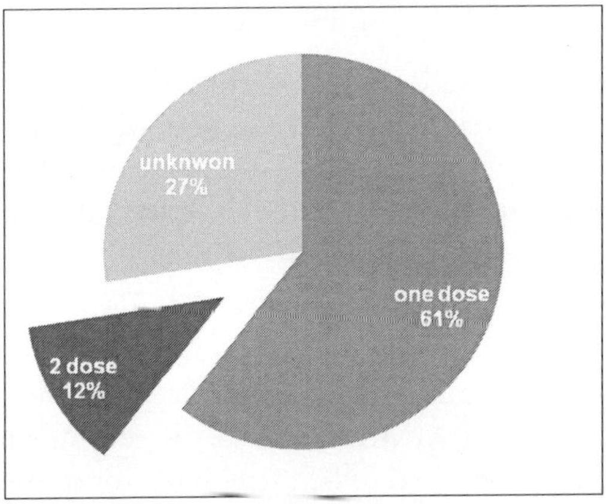

Fig. 2: Immunization Status of Affected Population Received Single and Double Doses, while about 27% of Affected Population was Unknown about their Immunization Status

This was clear when we reviewed the history of MMR vaccine since MMR vaccine was introduced to the EPI in 1988 as a single dose at 15 month of age (see Table 2). Two campaigns of MMR were performed, the first one in 17 Sep. 2005 for those born between (1983–1999) which targeted the primary and secondary schools, and university teachers and student. The second campaign targeted children born from July 1st, 2007 and after. This means that every child born from July 1st, 2007 and after was expected to be protected by 2 dose of MMR. The persons affected by the Bait Kahel mumps outbreak in the 9–14 years age group received only a single dose of MMR Jeryl Lynn vaccine, similar to the age group (5–16 years) who were affected in a previous outbreak in Gaza strip in 2013–2014 and received also a single dose of MMR. All household, school, college, and close contacts were followed to detect any undiagnosed and unreported cases. 62 cases were laboratory diagnosed and 619 clinically diagnosed from the beginning of outbreak on May 20th 2015 to January 16th January 2016. In 60% of cases, no medical care for parotid is and fever was sought, since people started to keep their children in home without seeking medical support because they perceived that there was nothing to be done, except giving their children acetaminophen as a pain killer and antipyretic in addition to supportive nutritional advice. The reporting of cases from schools depended on absence days of children as an indicator to call the family to ask about their children's absence. About 40% of cases were seen by a medical practitioner at the time of parotitis and complications included 14 cases of meningitis and 1 case of pancreatitis which required hospitalization. Outbreak continued although with less intensity till the date of writing of this report.

Control measures taken are included: alerting medical services providers, actively contacting children in medical practices who were not up to date with MMR vaccine by notification of families, in addition to alerting schools and health care providers through letters, media, and religious leaders.

4. CONCLUSIONS

In conclusion, this outbreak affected a specific group mainly those who received only one dose of MMR vaccine. It is recommended that high vaccination coverage is required to be maintained for second doses.

REFERENCES

[1] Ghuneim, N. and Dheir, M. (2015). The ongoing outbreak of mumps affecting all age groups among Gazans, occupied Palestinian territories 2013. *International Research Journal of Medicine and Medical Sciences* 3: 26–29.

[2] Hindiyeh, M.Y., Aboudy, Y., Wohoush, M., Shulman, L.M., Ram, D., Levin, T., Frank, T., Riccardo, F., Khalili, M., Sawalha, E.S., Obeidi, M., Sabatinelli, G., Grossman, Z. and Mendleson, E. (2009). Characterization of large mumps outbreak among vaccinated Palestinian refugees. *J Clin Microbiol* 47: 650–655.

[3] MOH (2016). Annual Health Report 2015. Ramallah: Ministry of Health, Government of Palestine, Ramallah, Palestine.

Vaccine Development and Immunization Schemes in Myanmar

Kyaw Phone Zaw[1*], Win Maw[2], Myo Khin[3], Hla Myat Mon[4] and Lei Win[1]

[1]National Analytical Laboratory, Department of Research and Innovation, Ministry of Education, Myanmar

[2]Myanmar Pharmaceutical Factory

[3]Department of Medical Research, Myanmar

[4]Department of Biotechnology, Yangon Technological University, Myanmar

*E-mail: kyawphonezaw2013@gmail.com

ABSTRACT: Vaccines have been shown as useful and important substances or medicines for prophylaxis of infectious diseases by decreasing disease outbreak and caused death. Despite several different kinds of vaccines which are produced by conventional methods such as MMR (Measles, Mumps, Rubella) and DPT (Diphtheria, Tetanus, Pertussis) are available for improving public health, new methods are needed to develop vaccines that induce strong and protective immune responses against specific infections. Today, researchers apply molecular biology and biotechnology approaches while developing new vaccines to overcome some limitations of conventional vaccines. For Myanmar, the Department of Medical Research and Myanmar Pharmaceutical Factory are the main organizations responsible for research and development of vaccines. The milestones of these two organizations in the 21st century is the successful local development of recombinant hepatitis B vaccine but production of conventional vaccines and anti-snake venom against viper and cobra of local species had been started for past decade. As multi years plan, expanded immunization program (EPI) has been carried out to immunize the whole country against preventable infectious diseases. A significant improvement was seen, according to data described by WHO, from an effective immunization program in Myanmar.

Keywords: Prophylaxis, MMR, DPT, Recombinant Hepatitis B Vaccine, Anti-Snake Venom, EPI.

1. INTRODUCTION

Vaccines are powerful tools not only in preventing incidence of infectious diseases but also contribute to significantly improve public health all over the world (Rebecca and Philip 2015). Since vaccines are considered the most cost efficient biological products for public health, today over 100 vaccines are available in different forms and formulations, so research and development in vaccinology may also be regarded as a major public concern. Many effective vaccines including live-attenuated vaccines or inactivated vaccines have been developed several years ago to induce host's immunity against several infections (Rebecca and Philip 2015). Due to some drawbacks of these vaccines, generation of DNA vaccines was introduced in medical research in the early 1990s with the help of molecular microbiology, recombinant DNA technology and biotechnology. With the improved understanding the etiology of certain infectious diseases and the emergence of new technologies, development of more vaccines may be possible (Jessica and Barry 2012). For Myanmar, the national vaccine production had been initiated, half of the century ago, exactly since 1957. Thus, it is justified to claim that Myanmar has a strong tradition in vaccine research and development for the past five decades. Myanmar Pharmaceutical Factory formerly known as Burma Pharmaceutical Industry (BPI) is considered the pioneer for national vaccine development and production. After its construction had been completed in 1957, BPI started production of 41 pharmaceuticals and 6 biological items. The substantial investments were made to satisfy the increasing demand for safer and more effective vaccines. For vaccine production, ministry of Health and Sport, the former name of the Ministry of Health (MoH), lunched immunization and health care programs to reduce outbreaks of some preventable diseases among people of different age groups.

This paper summarizes what researchers are doing to produce effective vaccines and how an expanded immunization program can be implemented for eradication and elimination of communicable diseases. The objective of this paper is to point out the national efforts on vaccine research and development and attempts on vaccination for reduction of mortality rates due to preventable communicable diseases.

2. ATTEMPTS ON VACCINE DEVELOPMENT

The following points represent brief descriptions of activities and development of national vaccine research and production in Myanmar.

2.1 Development of First Set of Vaccines

Communicable diseases like smallpox, cholera, plague and typhoid caused by microorganisms appeared to be a nightmare with dramatic psychological impact on community. One of the major contributions in microbiology and immunology is the development of vaccines to combat such bacteria and viruses. The first vaccines were created by weakened virus (*e.g.* Smallpox, Rabies) or killed or inactivated bacteria (*e.g.* pertussis) leading to induction of specific protective immune responses (Ruth and Tamar 2003). In the early time, the transfer of live-attenuated virus from human to human or animal to human was planned (Jessica and Barry 2012), but at the time of Louis Pasteur, artificially weakened pathogens were used as vaccines because mammalian cell culture techniques were established and pathogenic microbes were propagated *in vitro* (Rebecca and Philip 2015). Vaccines derived from these methods are recognized as conventional or traditional vaccines. As for Myanmar, between the year 1960–70, freeze dried form of smallpox vaccines, cholera vaccines, phenol inactivated liquid form as well as beta-propiolactone treated form of rabies vaccines and anti-venoms for passive immunization against both local viper and cobra species were developed by the BPI. The production and quality control were carried out according to the WHO guidelines including safety, efficacy and acceptable quality. People solely relied on BPI facilities and became confident in the national vaccine production technology. So, endemic and epidemic diseases such as smallpox, cholera, plague and typhoid had been prevented by conventional vaccines locally produced by the BPI. In addition, from the year 2006 to 2010, tissue culture based rabies vaccine was introduced to replace sheep brain vaccine. The first batch was produced in 2010. From the beginning of the production, depending on the annual demands of the MoH, the BPI produced and supplied 2.2 million doses vaccines of prophylactic as well as therapeutic (anti tetanus serum, anti-diphtheria serum) to hospitals and medical stores.

2.2 Development of Second Set of Vaccines

Efforts were made to avoid drawbacks of both live and inactivated vaccines which resulted in development of subunit vaccines for certain infectious diseases such as *Tetanus Toxoid (TT)* and diphtheria toxoid. Advances in biotechnology and molecular biology approaches enabled development of recombinant vaccines for some communicable diseases like hepatitis B and veterinary pathogens. These vaccines include toxic components of pathogenic microbes which are required to specifically stimulate host immunity against infective organisms. These vaccines are termed second generation vaccines and people all over the world have been using for a long time. In Myanmar, development and use of tetanus toxoid and diphtheria toxoid by the BPI were introduced in 1970. The combination of these two toxoid vaccines and Pertussis vaccines as (DPT) helped to cover the children from nationwide. Similarly, the Department of Medical Research (DMR), another responsible organization for vaccine development in Myanmar, expanded its research activities on various aspects of viral diseases. The invaluable achievement of the DMR during this decade is the development of vaccines to protect against hepatitis B virus (HBV). At first, working together with WHO and UNDP, researchers in DMR tried to produce plasma derived hepatitis B vaccines in a small scale. Later, recombinant hepatitis B vaccine was produced in 2004 with the aid of Republic of Korea after molecular genetics research on hepatitis viruses was established (Kyi 2013). Comparative study showed that in order to obtain, 225 mg of HB antigen, the required amount for 1000,000 vaccine dosages, one needs 35 liters of HBV infected blood plasma, whereas 5 gm of purified HB antigen produced from a single ampoule of recombinant yeast cell bank are enough to generate 5000,000 1000,000 vaccine dosages and both vaccines have similar immunologic capacity and protective efficacy. This clearly indicates that using biotechnology to produce recombinant HB vaccines with the WHO GMP acceptable quality is the method of choice to scale up the vaccine to the commercial level (Aung *et al.,* 2008, 2010). Moreover, researchers in the DMR identified the optimum conditions for vaccine production and quality control. For confirmation of safety and efficacy of both the plasma derived and recombinant HBV vaccines, clinical trials were conducted in 2006 and 2007, then successful technology transfer to the BPI for large scale production was carried out. The locally developed recombinant HBV vaccine in Myanmar will play an important role in preventing new infections.[4] Some of the ongoing research resulted in developing vaccines for rotaviruses and cholera.

2.3 Expanded Program on Immunization (EPI)

The coupling of vaccine development and immunization programs can help in reducing incidence of vaccine preventable diseases. In Myanmar, the EPI was implemented since the compound vaccines such as BCG, DPT vaccines were developed. By the year 1987, measles and polio vaccines were integrated into the EPI for young children. Since, vaccination is recognized as essential strategy for diseases control and reduction of mortality rates, supplementary immunization activities such as the National Immunization Days for polio and *Japanese encephalitis (JE)* eradiation, tetanus elimination in pregnant women and children under six month old were conducted. In addition, special programs of vaccination have been provided during favorable seasons in some townships. The significant improvement can be seen in prevention of some important infectious diseases as a result of implementing strong immunization programs and collaboration with international NGOs (Anonymous 2015). According to the WHO and UNICEF estimations, the coverage of Diphtheria-Pertussis-Tetanus (DPT) and *Haemophilius Influenza* B and HBV compound vaccines in children reached more than 80% while oral polio vaccine coverage reached about 89% (Anonymous 2017).

3. DISCUSSION

Vaccination has proven to be the most efficient, cost effective mean for preventing a wide variety of infectious diseases. Myanmar has good momentum to eradicate viral and bacterial diseases through development of first and second generation vaccines. A memorable milestone in our history is the development of both plasma-derived and recombinant HBV vaccines. A recent study showed that the production capacity of recombinant HBV vaccine is ten times higher than that of the plasma-derived hepatitis one which makes the recombinant vaccine more economic and easily scalable to fulfill the national needs with high quality and safety (Aung *et al.,* 2008, 2010). Manufacturing some vaccines had not been carried out due to either the decline in the prevalence of some diseases or the donation of some vaccines by the INGOs and the WHO. In addition, researchers in Myanmar have been doing ongoing research for production rotaviruses and cholera vaccines (Anonymous 2015). In addition, EPI implemented in Myanmar is strong and effective for eradication and elimination of epidemic and endemic diseases nationwide. Monitoring and evaluation of the immunization programs have been undertaken to increase the coverage rate and subsequently increase response to vaccination (Anonymous 2015).

4. SUMMARY

In summary, in Myanmar the first vaccines against plague and typhoid and two kinds of toxoid vaccines for tetanus and diphtheria were produced in BPI many years ago. Similarly, two different forms of HBV vaccines namely plasma-derived recombinant were developed by the DMR.[4] The results from a comparative study of the plasma-derived and the recombinant HBV vaccines and the quality assurance testing was pointed out. Local production of HBV vaccines can support combating liver diseases caused by the viral infection. In combination with vaccine research and development, implementation of strong and effective EPI and its achievements were highlighted.

ACKNOWLEDGEMENTS

The support by the Department of Research and Innovation is fully acknowledged. The author would like to express gratitude to the Director General, the Deputy Director General, the Directors and Deputy Directors for their guidance and kind encouragement to accomplish this paper. He is also indebted to all co-authors for their support and helpful discussions.

REFERENCES

[1] Anonymous (2015). Expanded Program on Immunization (EPI): Multi Year Plan, Myanmar Immunization Programme. Department of Health, The Republic of the Union of Myanmar, cMYP 2012–2016, pp. 1–34.
http://www.nationalplanningcycles.org/Myanmar/cmpy-2012-2016-12-nov-11-pdf

[2] Anonymous (2017). EPI Fact Sheet. Regional Office for South East Asia, World Health Organization. SEARO/FGL/IVD http://www.searo.who.int/entity/immunization/data/myanmar-2017.pdf?ua-1

[3] Aung, W. *et al.* (2008). Quality assurance of the recombinant Hepatitis B vaccine produced at the GMP standard Hepatitis B Plant, DMR. *The Myanmar Health Sciences Research Journal* 20: 33–38.

[4] Aung, W. *et al.* (2010). Production, quality control and immune response of the plasma-derived and the yeast-derived recombinant Hepatitis B vaccines locally developed at the Hepatitis B vaccines Plant, DMR (LM): Comparative study. *The Myanmar Health Sciences Research Journal* 20: 105–111.

[5] Jessica, O.J. and Barry, B. (2012). Vaccine Process Technology. *J Biotechnol Bioeng* 109: 1443–1460.

[6] Kyi, K.P. (2013). Viral Hepatitis. Further development of medical research in Myanmar (1987–2011). DMR Bulletin, pp. 199–202.

[7] Mariana *et al.* (2010). DNA vaccines for targeting bacterial infections. *Expert Rev Vaccines* 9: 747–763.

[8] Rebecca, J.L. and Philip, R.J. (2015). Emerging vaccine technologies. *Vaccines* 3: 429–447.

[9] Ruth, A. and Tamar, B.Y. (2003). Old and New Vaccine Approaches. *International Immunopharmacology,* 3: 1195–1204.

Measles Outbreak in 2013 Sri Lanka: Lessons Learnt for Global Measles Elimination Programme

D. Wickramasinghe[1], S.B. Agampodi[2] and D. Vidanagama[3]

[1,3]Department of Microbiology, Teaching Hospital Karapitiya, Karapitiya

[2]Department of Community Medicine, Faculty of Medicine, University of Rajarata, Anuradhapura

[1]E-mail: dwickw2@yahoo.co.uk; dhampara@gmail.com

ABSTRACT: Sri Lanka received the measles elimination status in 2012–13, 28 years after introduction of measles containing vaccine to Sri Lankan expanded programme of immunization (EPI) in 1984. In year 2013, Sri Lanka experienced an outbreak of measles with 3995 reported cases, the largest outbreak in Sri Lanka since initiation of two-dose vaccination schedule in 2002. Most severely affected districts were the Galle and Anuradhapura with confirmed cases. In this report we are examining the further evidence of 2013 outbreak of measles from the Galle district. This study was conducted in the teaching hospital Karapitiya from February 2013 to February 2014. All clinically suspected patients of measles admitted to pediatric and medical wards were initially included in the investigation. Disease confirmation was done at Medical Research Institute, Colombo. A total of 285 measles cases were admitted which included 109 (38.2%) females and 176 (61.8%) males. Median duration of symptoms on admission was 3 days. Distribution of cases by months showed that the peak of the outbreak was in July 2013. Age distribution of measles cases during the outbreak showed that the outbreak was exclusively among infants less than 12 months of age during the first month and there was a gradual increase of cases from other age groups starting from the second month. As expected, majority of the cases were from Galle district (237, 83.2%) followed by Matara (43, 15.1%) and Hambantota (5, 1.85%). Our analysis clearly shows that the initial outbreak of measles in the study population was among unvaccinated infants. The change of vaccine schedule in 2012 was done to include MMR (measles, mumps and rubella) vaccine to the EPI schedule, to achieve elimination of congenital rubella syndrome and complications of mumps. The decision was taken after achieving measles elimination goals and careful evaluation of current status of all three diseases. However, this outbreak of measles shows that maintaining disease elimination status is always a challenge.

Keywords: Measles Outbreak, EPI, Cohort, Vaccination, Infant Immunization.

1. INTRODUCTION

Sri Lanka received the measles elimination status in 2012, 28 years after introduction of measles containing vaccine to Sri Lankan ***Expanded Programme of Immunization (EPI)*** in 1984. In year 2013, Sri Lanka experienced an outbreak of measles with 3995 reported cases, the largest outbreak in Sri Lanka, since introduction of two-dose vaccination in 2002 (Dahanayaka *et al.*, 2015). Despite being one of the most important public health issues in last decade, scientific investigation into 2013 outbreak of measles in Sri Lanka is rather scattered and less explored. The only published article using confirmed cases was from Anuradhapura district with 32 confirmed cases and it attribute the outbreak to the change of vaccination schedule, which was was done to include ***MMR (Measles, Mumps and Rubella)*** vaccine to the EPI schedule, to achieve elimination of congenital rubella syndrome and complications of mumps. However, age disaggregated analysis of confirmed cases is not available yet in published literature. Galle district had one of the highest incidence of measles during 2013 outbreak of measles with an incidence around 25/100,000 population. We presented here further evidence of 2013 outbreak of measles from Galle district.

2. MATERIALS AND METHODS

This study was conducted in the ***Teaching Hospital Karapitiya (THK)*** in Galle, Sri Lanka from February 2013 to February 2014. All clinically suspected patients of measles admitted to pediatric and medical wards were initially included in the investigation. Disease confirmation was done at Medical Research Institute, Colombo. Only the confirmed cases of measles were included in this analysis. A total of 285 measles cases were admitted to THK from April 2013 to February 2014. These included 109 (38.2%) females and 176 (61.8%) males and the average duration of symptoms on admission was observed in 3 days. Distribution of cases was also analyzed by the months to evaluate the seasonal prevalence of the outbreak. Age categorization was done according to the immunization cohorts, which include infants as follows:

- **Cohort-I** : less than 6 months (probably having maternal antibodies)
- **Cohort-II** : 6–8 months of age (not suitable for immunization)
- **Cohort-III** : 9–12 months (vaccinated as previous schedule before 2012)
- **Cohort-IV** : 1–12 years (children received two doses schedule)
- **Cohort-V** : 13–28 years (cohort received single dose schedule) and
- **Cohort-VI** : more than 28 years (unvaccinated cohort).

3. RESULTS

3.1 Sri Lanka during 2013 Outbreak

3.1.1 *Measles Cases Admitted to Teaching Hospital Karapitiya (THK)*

A total of 285 measles cases were admitted to THK from April 2013 to February 2014. These included 109 (38.2%) females and 176 (61.8%) males. Median duration of symptoms on admission was observed in 3 days. Distribution of cases by months showed that the peak of the outbreak was in July 2013 (see Figure 1).

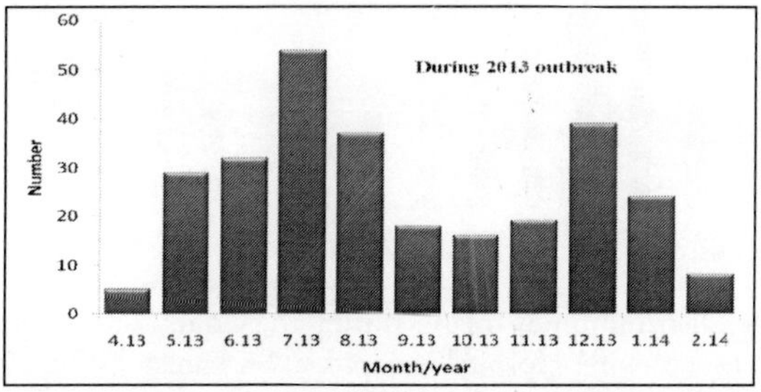

Fig. 1: Epidemic Curve of Measeles Cases Admitted to Teaching Hospital Karapitiya, Galle, Sri Lanka during 2013 Outbreak

3.1.2 *Age Distribution of Measles Cases during 2013 Outbreak*

Age categorization was done among the confirmed cases according to the immunization cohorts with special reference to the infants, 6 cohorts were formed as mentioned in the materials and methods. In 2013 outbreak, it was observed that unvaccinated cohort-I and II accounted for 32.3% of the cases followed by cohort-III 23%, which had been vaccinated according to the previous schedule before 2012 (see Figure 2). Group with the two dose schedule was the least affected (3.9%).

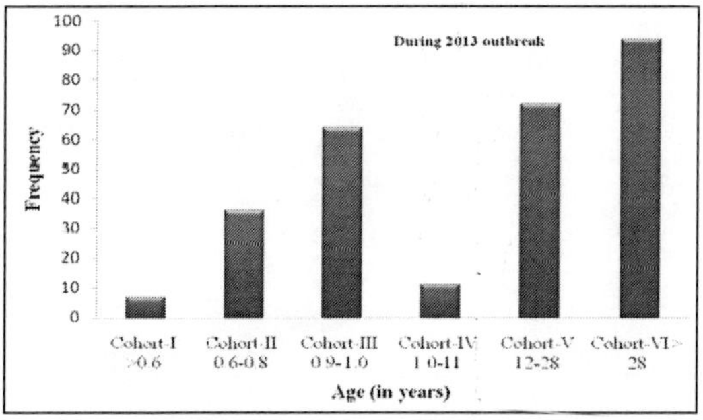

Fig. 2: Age Distribution of Measeles Cases Admitted to Teaching Hospital Karapitiya, Sri Lanka during 2013 Outbreak

3.2 Distribution of Infants during the Course of Measles Epidemic

Age distribution of measles cases during the outbreak showed that the outbreak was exclusively among infants less than 12 months of age during the first month and there was a gradual increase of cases from other age groups starting from the second month (see Figure 3).

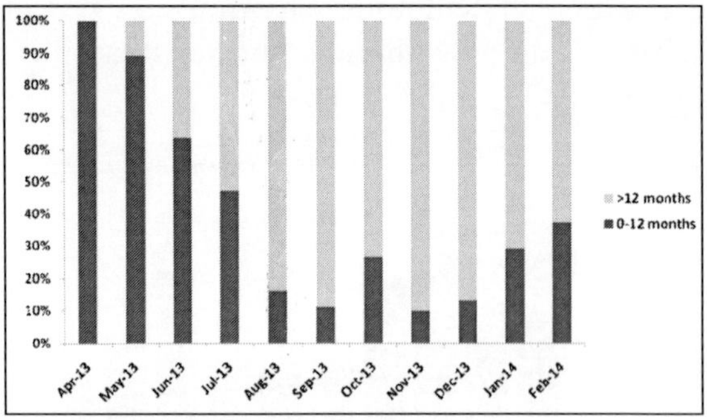

Fig. 3: Percentage Distribution of Infants during the Course of Epidemic of Measeles Cases Admitted to Teaching Hospital Karapitiya, Sri Lanka during 2013 Outbreak

3.3 Geographical Distribution of Reported Cases of Measles in 2013

As expected, majority of the cases were from Galle district (237, 83.2%) followed by Matara (43, 15.1%) and Hambantota (5, 1.85%). Geographical distribution of reported cases showed that most of the cases admitted were from Hikkaduwa, Baddegama, Habaraduwa, Akmeemana and Galle Fort (see Figure 4). The measles incidence in MOH divisions

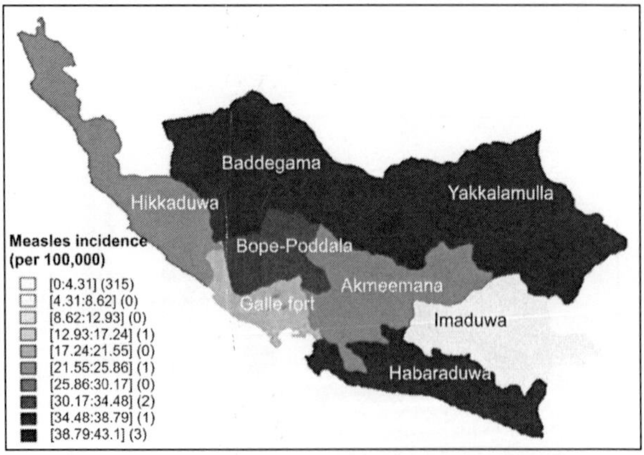

Fig. 4: Incidence of Measles in Medical Officers of Health Areas Surrounding Teaching Hospital Karapitiya

surrounding the hospital (draining areas to study setting) was calculated to identify the geographical distribution of disease.

4. DISCUSSION AND CONCLUSIONS

Our analysis clearly shows that the initial outbreak of measles in the study population was among unvaccinated infants, who would have received measles vaccine if the vaccine schedule was not changed (Mahipala 2015). Later, the outbreak was mainly among the unvaccinated adult cohort. The same was observed in Anuradhapura district, based on clinically suspected cases and our study confirmed the previous observation. As argued in the previous papers, infants receive passive immunity against measles from mother. If the mother had vaccine derived immunity, the infants will have low level of immunity. The passive immunity from mother starts declining at around five to nine months and infants become susceptible to measles thereafter (Sato *et al.,* 1979). Before 2012, measles was given at nine months (WHO 1982) and in the revised schedule it was at 12 months. The schedule revision added a large cohort of susceptible infants to the population. This added susceptible cohort might have contributed to crossing the population heard immunity level, igniting an outbreak. The change of vaccine schedule in 2012 was done to include MMR ***(measles, mumps and rubella)*** vaccine to the EPI schedule, to achieve elimination of congenital rubella syndrome and complications of mumps. The decision was taken after achieving measles elimination goals and careful evaluation of current status of all three diseases. However, this outbreak of measles shows that maintaining disease elimination status is always a challenge, very similar to achieving it. The health services in the Sri Lanka by Ministry of Health have taken steps to revise the EPI schedule from 1st April 2015. The new schedule will provide MMR vaccination at nine months and administer the Live Japanese Encephalitis vaccine at twelve months.

REFERENCES

[1] Dahanayaka N.J., Pahalagamage S., Ganegama R.M., Weerawansa P. and Agampodi S.B. (2015). The 2013 measles outbreak in Sri Lanka: experience from a rural district and implications for measles elimination goals. *Infect Dis Poverty,* 4: 51.

[2] Sato H., Albrecht P., Reynolds D.W., Stagno S. and Ennis F.A. (1979). Transfer of measles, mumps and rubella antibodies from mother to infant. Its

effect on measles, mumps and rubella immunization. *Am J Dis Child,* 133: 1240–1243.

[3] WHO (1982). World Health Organization-The optimal age for measles immunization. *Wkly Epidemiol Rec.,* 57: 89–91.

[4] Mahipala P.G. (2015). Change of the national immunization schedule: MMR, LJE vaccination. Circular from The Ministry of Health and Indigenous Medicine of Sri Lanka dated 18/03/2015 of reference My No. EPI/14/2015.

Section 2

Vaccine Development Strategies

Innovation and Technology Development in Vaccine Production in Vietnam

Do Tuan Dat[1], Nguyen Thu Van[1], Vu Hong Nga[1], Dang Duc Anh[2] and Le Quynh Mai[2]

[1]D&B Hoovars, Company for Vaccine and Biological Production No. 1, Hanoi, Vietnam

[2]National Institute of Hygiene and Epidemiology (NIHE), Yersin Street, Hanoi, Vietnam

E-mail: ltqm@nihe.org.vn; lom9@hotmail.com

ABSTRACT: Recent advances in vaccine technology arising from the application of genetic engineering, cell culture, and recombinant protein and conjugation techniques are now providing an opportunity to control infectious diseases. Applying such new technology improves purity, safety and effectiveness and decreases the costs of production. We focus in this paper on how new effective vaccines such as recombinant hepatitis B, inactivated hepatitis A, mouse brain derived Japanese encephalitis, oral cholera, oral live attenuated poliomyelitis vaccine, measles, diphtheria, tetanus, pertussis, BCG, typhoid Vi polysaccharide vaccine, rotavirus and other vaccines could be developed and produced in Vietnam. This requires investment from the government for technological innovation, research and development, production and clinical trials of vaccines in order to meet the demand of the country.

Keywords: Vaccine, Production Technology, Inactivation, Recombinant, Live Attenuated, Vietnam.

1. INTRODUCTION

One of the ground breaking discoveries of the 20th Century is the vaccine, as an arsenal for fighting against the infectious diseases. Vaccination is known to be an effective measure for public health tools emphasized in the global agenda of United Nations-Sustainable developmental Goals (SDGs). The United nations recognize the crisis of child mortality (SDG-4) and improvement of maternal health (SDG-5) in developing countries (United Nations 2016). The new WHO Global Action Plan and Monitoring Framework for the Prevention and Control of non-communicable diseases (NCDs) create a robust global architecture and vaccination as a key pillar in fighting against NCDs (Raw and Higashi 1984). There has been a significant advancement made in developing, introducing and expanding the global vaccine reach, including vaccine for the eradication of polio and reduction in deaths caused by vaccine-preventable diseases like Diphtheria, Measles, Neonatal tetanus, Pertussis (Morales *et al.,* 2018, Raw and Higashi 1984, Jadhav *et al.,* 2014).

In developing countries, infectious diseases are causing big outbreaks and account for around half of all deaths of which about 90% of these mortalities related to diarrheal and respiratory diseases. Further, these countries, where economic development is lacking, priority must be given to primary healthcare and establishment of sustainable healthcare delivery system. Thus, introducing a new vaccine (including a new generation vaccine) in a developing country may face several financial and logistic challenges, as a result several vaccines which were previously used are being replaced with newer generation vaccines in the developed world (*e.g.* whole-cell Pertussis vaccine being replaced by acellular Pertussis vaccine) but continue to be use in developing countries due to their low cost (Morales *et al.,* 2018, Raw and Higashi 1984, Jadhav *et al.,* 2014, Pagliusi *et al.,* 2013). In Vietnam, the earlier vaccine studies were operated in Pasteur Institutions in Saigon, Nha Trang and Dalat, which was led by Dr. Alexandre Yersin (1890–1943) and since 1960, several vaccines have been administered such as smallpox, BCG, oral polio and tetanus toxoid. Mass vaccination campaigns also have been carried out (UNICEF 2009). Vietnam launched its Expanded Program on Immunization (EPI) in 1981 based on the WHO recommendation with a view to protect all eligible children against six childhood diseases (Tuberculosis, Diphtheria, Pertussis, Measles, Tetanus, Polio Myelitis), and most of them (BCG-DPT and OPV) were local vaccines (Jit *et al.,* 2015). Then, in the past twenty years, the vaccine manufacturers achieved significant development and approached to the policy of the government and Ministry of Health (MoH) "self-reliant local production of vaccine" that conferred immunity against more than 10 dangerous infectious diseases and provided a greatest benefit for children in Vietnam through the EPI program. Vietnam is among the countries which have certification of polio elimination in 2000 and of maternal and neonatal tetanus in 2005, and this reflects success of the EPI program and science achievements of vaccine production (UNICEF 2009). Recently, outbreaks of emerging infectious diseases have been occurring (SARS-CoV, avian influenza A/H5N1) as well as shortage in essential and pentavalant vaccines (Rabies, DPT-HibB-IPV) in Vietnam provided a timely reminder of the vaccine supply and the possibility of disrupting access to vaccines against most serious and common diseases. The application of new technologies to the assessment, development and production of vaccines has the potential to provide adequate essential vaccines according to public health demand and enable the introduction of new vaccines in Vietnam. However, introducing the new technologies or innovation for vaccine productions in developing countries may face several financial and logistical challenges (MacLennan 2013, Nguyen *et al.,* 2005).

Vietnam is achieving success as a middle-income country since 2011 however, the health system has faced the challenge of the widespread withdrawal of external funding for continuing health care activities. Further, an extraordinary challenge is buying vaccines with significantly higher prices than low-income countries which have access to international support to buy vaccines. Thus, innovation and technological development in vaccine production are vital requirements for reaching 'self-sufficiency at least in the essential vaccines against emerging and common diseases for Vietnamese' (Pagliusi *et al.,* 2013, MacLennan 2013). Likely some countries such as Brazil, India, Cuba and Indonesia, Vietnam has invested in research for the purpose of large-scale vaccine manufacturing. In the present paper we summarize the current situation of vaccine manufactures and innovative trend of technologies in vaccine development in Vietnam.

2. METHODS AND METHODS

We reviewed twenty state-scientific projects on vaccine development in the period from 1991 to 2015 as well as approached key Government circulars/decisions that were issued by the MoH and Ministry of Science and Technology (MOST).

3. VACCINE MANUFACTURING IN VIETNAM

3.1 Current Status of Vaccine Manufacturing

Vietnam is one of just a few countries in the region that can produce own vaccines by local vaccine manufacturing facilities. Currently, there are four state-owned vaccine manufacturers, two located in Hanoi (northern) and two in Nha Trang (Central) and Dalat (Highland) (see Figure 1).

The names of these companies are:

- Company for Vaccine and Biological Production No. 1 (**VABIOTECH**), Hanoi.

- Center for Research and Production of Vaccines and Medico-Biological products, Hanoi (**POLYVAC**).
- Institute of Vaccines and Medico-Biological Products, Nha Trang (**IVAC**).
- Company for Vaccine Production Pasteur, Dalat (**DAVAC**).

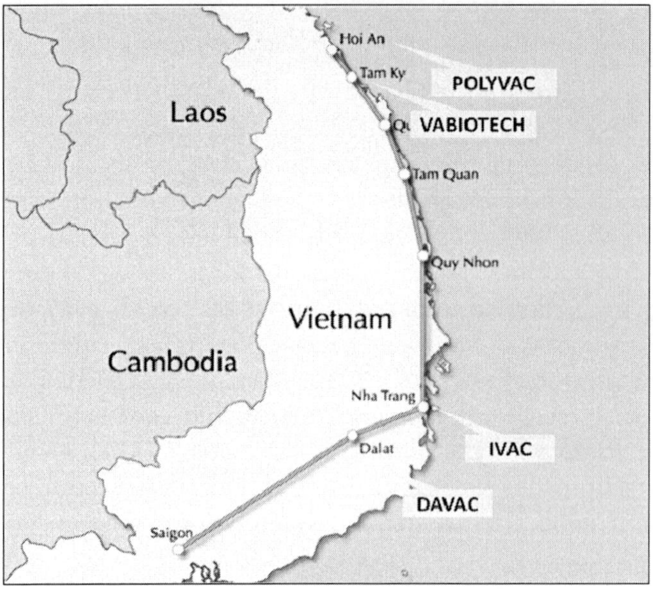

Fig. 1: Four State-Owned Vaccine Manufacturers in Vietnam, Two Located in Hanoi (POLYVAC and VABIOTECH), one in Nha Trang (IVAC) and another One in Dalat (DAVAC)

The two enterprises located in Hanoi were originally integrated within the National Institute of Hygiene and Epidemiology, Hanoi (NIHE), and then subsequently became independent enterprises in 1994 (POLYVAC) and 2007 (VABIOTECH), respectively. Each of the enterprises is now parastatal with 50% publically traded stocks/shares with the government retaining at least 50% ownership. The four manufactures are members of the ***DCVMN (Developing Countries Vaccine Manufacturing Network)*** which continues to facilitate training opportunities and provides support for technology transfer.

3.2 Vaccine Production Capacities

Vietnam already manufactures 11 out of 12 vaccines used in the ***National Expanded Program on Immunization (NEPI)*** for children, including vaccines against Tuberculosis, Diphtheria, Pertussis, Tetanus, Hepatitis B, Measles, Polio, Japanese B encephalitis, Cholera, Typhoid, Rubella and *Haemophilus influenza* Type b (Hib) (see Table 1). In Vietnam, about 1.7 million children are born every year and they all received free vaccination under the NEPI program. The NEPI program uses approximately 35–40 million doses a year, comprising approximately 92% of all vaccines used in the country (see Table 2).

Table 1: Vaccination Schedule of the Vietnam *National Expanded Program on Immunization* (NEPI) for year 2016

Vaccines	*Birth*	*2M*	*3M*	*4M*	*9M*	*18M*
BCG	×					
Hepatitis B	×					
OPV		×	×	×		
DPT-Hepatitis B-Hib		×	×	×		
Measles					×	
Measles-rubella						×
DPT						×
Japanese Encephalitis	Two doses in the first year at 1-2 weeks interval, and 3rd dose at 1 year interval					
Typhoid (in high risk areas)	One dose for 3–10 years old					
Cholera (in high risk areas)	Two doses at 1 month interval for 2–5 years old					
Tetanus toxoid (in high risk areas)	Pregnant women or child bearing age women					

Table 2: Estimated Production Capacity of Vaccines Produced by Vietnam State-Owned Enterprises for the Year 2016

Manu-facturer	*Vaccine*	*Current Status*	*Capacity/ Doses (in mL)*
POLYVAC	Measles		7.5
	Measles-Rubella	Through technology transfer from KDSV, Japan. Licensed since 2017.	7.5
	Rotavirus	With support from USCDC, WHO, MoH; licensed since 2012	4.0
	tOPV	Through technology transfer from Soviet Union Licensed in Vietnam since 1960	40

Manu-facturer	*Vaccine*	*Current Status*	*Capacity/ Doses (in mL)*
	bOPV	In process changing from tOPV to bOPV. Scheduled for production in 2017	40
	IPV	Sabin strain, under Phase-2 trial	Lab. scale
IVAC	DTP		15
	BCG		8.0
	TT		20
	Td		10
	Seasonal influenza TIV	Completed Ph1 clinical trial; Ph2 planning ongoing	
VA-BIOTECH	Hepatitis B	Recombivax formulation licensed since 2001	20
	Hepatitis A	Licensed since 2003	0.3
	JEV	Licensed and produced in SMB, since 1997	6.0
	JEV	Vero-grown, Completed Phase-1 clinical trial, Phase-2 ongoing	NA
	Oral cholera		8–10
	Rabies vaccine (vero-grown)	Clinical trials were planned in 2017	

4. TRENDS IN VACCINE INNOVATION AND DEVELOPMENT IN VIETNAM

Technologies for production of individual vaccines and combination vaccines are established in Vietnam and most of them are safe, effective and used in national immunization program. The Vietnamese healthcare system is formed by government and local public entities and is supported by 0.9% of the *Gross Domestic Product (GDP)* of the country. However, the preventive medicine system is widely distributed from central level to local level with routine surveillance as well as the activities of the NEPI. Vietnam is one of 25 countries in the world that supplies most of vaccines to support NEPI through domestic manufacturing. In addition, Vietnam has a long history of high quality vaccine production for exporting. Recently, all of Vietnamese manufactures became members of DCVMN which opens up opportunities for co-development of products, technology transfer and delivery of specific service or products.

4.1 Target Diseases for Upcoming Vaccine Development in Vietnam

Unlike developing countries where development and deployment of vaccines to protect against infectious diseases is a priority, the impact of NCDs in Vietnam is raising rapidly, and research on developing vaccines with potential to prevent chronic or cancer diseases is part of the national strategy for vaccine development. According to WHO recommendation, several important live-saving vaccines have become available in recent years, and a number of additional advanced or improved vaccines of public health importance are under consideration for the vaccine development strategy in Vietnam. Based on the magnitude of diseases and its impact on health and diseases burden data collected from regular surveillance, the National Institute of Hygiene and Epidemiology have analyzed and provided a set of priorities to target the diseases by the vaccine (see Table 3). Further, in order to sustain the NEPI's achievements, some new additional vaccines have been added for strengthening both the immune-zation program and health care system in Vietnam (see Table 3).

Table 3: Expected Vaccine for Innovation and Development in Vietnam

Upcoming vaccines of public health requirement	
Vaccine for NEPI	*Vaccine for Targeted Diseases*
Rotavirus (oral)	Malaria (RTS, S)
Pneumococcal conjugate (10 and 13 valent)	Dengue
Improved Japanese encephalitis (cell-based)	Human Papillomavirus (HPV)
Typhoid Vi conjugate	Pandemic influenza
Meningococcal (Monovalent, Tetra and Pentavalent conjugate)	Seasonal influenza (trivalent)
Tuberculosis (New generation)	Rabies (cell-based)
Monovalent and bivalent polio (OPV/IPV)	Enteroviruses (inactivated)
Universal Hepatitis B and Heamophilus influenza B (Hib conjugate)	Varicella
Combination 6 in 1 (D-T-aP-HepB-Hib-IPV)	

4.2 Inovation and Technology Application for Vaccine Development and Production in Vietnam

Vaccines are among the most cost-effective health intervention means in the history. Each year, vaccines save 2.5 million lives worldwide, yet 1.7 million children still die annually from vaccin-preventalbe diseases. Vietnam is working to realize life-saving benefits of vaccines and reduced the number of deaths through its NEPI program. Due to the success of the local vaccine manufacturers and in order to promote self-reliance and provide affordable supply for its own population, the Vietnamese Government has made a policy priority to accelerate production of inovative vaccines. Several advisory committees have played a role in recommending and promoting innovative technology in vaccine development. Recently, the Vietnamese Government's officials support vaccine manufactures (*i.e.* NIHE, IVAC, VABIOTECH *etc.*) to implement research and development (R&D) through scientific state projects with allocated commitment of funding. Additionally, the WHO and other international organizations like US-CDC, PATH, JICA have also provided financial and technical support for developing new vaccines such as MR, Pandemic influenza H5N1/H1N1pdm09, Trivalent seasonal influenza (TIV) (Nguyen *et al.*, d-f, Do *et al.*, 2009).

Innovation and development of technologies in vaccine manufacturing in Vietnam includes two trends. First, sustaining the traditional manufacturing processes with further development focusing on improving stability (*e.g.* novel excipients, novel adjuvants *etc.*), updating formulation (*e.g.* combination and recombinant vaccines), Purification techniques (e.g. Membrane adsorption, Precipitaiton), that resutls in increasing efficacy, cost-effective and convenient storages (see Table 4). Second,

Table 4: Inovative Technologies for Traditional Manufacturing Processes

Vaccines	*Used Technologies*	*Inovative Technologies*
Hepatitis B	Serum-based	Recombinant
Japaneses Encephalitis	Inactivated suckling mouse brains derived	Inactivated Vero cells-based
Oral Cholera (OCV)	Inactivated whole cells	
Hepatitis A	Inactivated primary cells based	Inactivated diploid cells based (MRC-5)
Diphtheria-Tetanus-Pertussis	Whole cell pertussis	Purified proteins of acellular pertussis
Bi-OPV	Live attenuated	Inactivated (IPV)

exploring new technologies such as cell-based, polysaccharide and conjugation, recombinant DNA, which act not only to improve vaccine manufacturing capacities, but also to develop new vaccines against common and dangerous diseases.

4.3 Roll of National Institution of Hygiene and Epidemiology (NIHE) in Vaccine Development in Vietnam

The NIHE is a major public health institute under the MoH. It oversees the prevention and control of epidemic and common diseaeses. Its functions include conducting scienctific research in epidemiology, medical microbiology, immunology, molecular biology and developing new vaccines and biologicals. Among history of vaccine development in Vietnam, NIHE was first institute to be involved in technology transfers as well as in promoting research and development of several vaccines like OPV, Hepatitits B, JE, Cholera, Hepatittis A and B. Other institutions like POLYVAC and VABIOTECH were then come into the existence after separation from NIHE, to provide them a greater autonomy and flexibility of commercial production of vaccine. The NIHE at present leading and co-ordinating the activities of NEPI, as well as conducts active surveillance of infectious diseases including vaccine-preventable diseases. The NIHE has also been involved in several longitudinal studies to support public health research on infectious diseases. The possibility of using data collected in surveillance system that functions consistently over time can be predictive trends of diseases in community, therefore, helpful to develop the strategies for appropriate use of a particular vaccine, specifically against outbreak of disease.

Combining new technologies along with continuous surveillance for vaccine-preventable diseases, NIHE has been able to select and provide appropriate antigenic materials and strains for vaccine development and manufacturing in affordable prices, which meets the requirements of public health.

5. CHALLENGES IN INNOVATION AND DEVELOPMENT OF TECHNOLOGY IN VACCINE PRODUCTIONS IN VIETNAM

Vaccines offer the most cost-effective approach to controlling disease, particularly in developing countries such as Vietnam. Innovation or introduction of new technologies for vaccine production is providing new biological which are safer and more immunogenic as well as cost effective.

However, the main challenges in innovation and development technology in vaccine manufacturing in Vietnam are both financial and strategic resources.

5.1 Decrease in Financial Investments

Since 2009, Vietnam's elevation to a lower-middle income country is a great achievement; however, the health system faces widespread withdrawal of external funding support for continuing health care activities, including reducing investment for innovation technology in vaccine development. The transition from internationally-supported programs to reliance on domestic Government resources and also creates a strong need for prioritizing targets and strategic planning. State budget spending on health has increased by 34.2% per year on average in the period of 2008–2013 higher than the increase in overall state budget recurrent spending. However, health care costs are also increasing thus priority of budget spending is not focused on vaccine development. To approach new technologies, the vaccine production units would require huge upgrading in their existing manufacturing facilities and constructing or re-constructing new infrastructures, but financing these plans has not yet been secured and a time frame for implementing these projects is thus unclear.

5.2 Inadequate Strategy for Vaccine Development

Since all of vaccine manufactures in Vietnam belongs to Government, thus, decision making regarding production, pricing and other developmental issues related to new products seeks directions MOH). The 'business plan' associating vaccine production is not considered or evaluated according to commercial markets, therefore, it has a negative impact on the amount of available recourses for Research and Development and for investment into new technologies in vaccine development.

6. CONCLUSION

Vaccines are determined as one of the most important public health achievements, especially when the benefit of childhood vaccines in reducing mortality are undeniable through the NEPI over the past 30 years in Vietnam. Recently, the urgent need to accelerate response to emerging threats makes vaccines more widely available and ready for quick deployment. Development of vaccines against NCDs has raised motivation of innovation in vaccine technology in Vietnam. Here, we reviewed current status of vaccine manufacturing in Vietnam and found that innovation or development technologies in vaccine productions is increasing in all vaccine manufactures in order to produce safer and more immunogenic vaccines in affordable costs. Although, supporting innovation and development technology is essential to achieve sustainable and profitable vaccines, however, manufacturers hope to gain more streamlined vaccine development requirements and effective investments from the government as well as international funding organizations.

ACKNOWLEDGMENT

We thank the colleagues from IVAC, POLYVAC, DAVAC and VABIOTECH for the helpful discussion and valuable suggestions. The authors alone are responsible for the views presented and expressed in this publication.

REFERENCES

[1] Dang, D.T. *et al.,* Application of advanced techniques to improve the vaccine production process for the Oral cholera vaccine. State Research Subject coded KY-01-03: Department of Science and Technology Information. Hanoi, Vietnam.

[2] Dang, D.T. *et al.,* Improving the technological process for manufacturing the oral cholera vaccine. State Pilot Production Project coded KHCN-11-DA4. Department of science and technology information, Hanoi, Vietnam.

[3] Do, T.D. *et al.,* Establish a technological process for manufacturing rabies vaccine on Vero cell culture in laboratory scale. State Research Subject coded KC.10.19 state/06-12, The Department of Science and Technology Information, Hanoi, Vietnam SDK: 2011-64-316/KQNC TTTTKHCN QG_8514.

[4] Do, T.D. *et al.,* Establish a technological process for manufacturing live attenuated dengue vaccine in the laboratory scale. State Research Subject coded KC10.12/11-15, The Department of Science and Technology Information, Hanoi, Vietnam SDK: 2014-64704/KQNC TTTTKHC NQG_10804.

[5] Do, T.N. *et al.,* Establish a technological process for manufacturing influenza A/H1N1 on primary monkey kidney cells and MDCK cells. Independent State Research Subject coded DTDL - 2009G/53, The Department of Science and Technology Information, Hanoi, Vietnam SDK: 2012-64-176/KQNC TTTTKHCNQG_9156.

[6] Hoa, L.K., Hiep, L.V. and Be, L.V. (2011). Development of pandemic influenza vaccine production capacity in Viet Nam. Vaccine 29: 34–36.

[7] Hong, N.V. *et al.,* Establish a technological process for manufacturing EV71 HFMD vaccine in the laboratory scale. State Research Subject coded KC.10. TN08/11-15, The Department of Science and Technology Information, Hanoi, Vietnam SDK: 2013-64-264/KQNC-TTKHC.

[8] Jadhav, S., Gautam, M. and Gairola, S. (2014). Role of vaccine manufacturers in developing countries towards global healthcare by providing quality vaccines at affordable prices. *Clin Microbiol Infect* 20: 37–44.

[9] Le, T.L. *et al.,* Assessment of the safety and the immunogenicity of the Oral Live Attenuated Rotavin- M1, vaccine for prevention of Diarrhea of children in Vietnam. . State Research Subject coded KC.10/06-10, The Department of Science and Technology Information, Hanoi, Vietnam.

[10] Le, T.L. *et al.,* Establish a technological process for manufacturing Oral Live Attenuated Rotavirus vaccine for prevention of diarrhea of children in Vietnam". State Research Subject coded KC.10.33/06-1, The Department of Science and Technology Information, Hanoi, Vietnam.

[11] Le, T.L. *et al.,* Improving the technological process for manufacturing the Oral Live Attenuated Rotavin-M1vaccine". State Pilot Production Project coded KC.10.DA07/11-15, The Department of Science and Technology Information, Hanoi, Vietnam.

[12] Lien, H.T.P. *et al.,* Improving technological process for manufacturing the Japanese encephalitis vaccine and the Diagnostic Kit for Japanese encephalitis virus and dengue. State Research Subject coded KY-01-04. Department of Science and Technology Information, Hanoi, Vietnam SDK: 96-64 -247.

[13] Lien, H.T.P. *et al.,* Improving technological process for manufacturing the Japanese Encephalitis vaccine. State Pilot Production Project coded KHCN-11-DA2. Department of Science and Technology Information, Hanoi, Vietnam.

[14] Lien, H.T.P. *et al.,* Research to replace Nakayama strain by Beijing-1 strain for manufacturing the Japanese encephalitis vaccine. State Research Subject coded KC-10-22, Department of Science and Technology Information. SDK 2006-64-324/KQNC TTTTKHCNQG_5983.

[15] Long, H.T. *et al.,* State Pilot Production Project coded KHCN11-DA1: Improving technological manufacturing process for human plasma derived hepatitis B vaccine at the scale of 500,000 children's doses/year. Department of science and technology information, Hanoi, Vietnam. http://www.scj.go.jp/en/sca/activities/conferences/conf_5_programs/pdf/5thas2van.pdf

[16] MacLennan, C.A. (2013). Vaccines for low-income countries. Semin Immunol 25: 114–123.

[17] Mark, J., Dang, T.T.H., Ingrid, F., Hoang, V.M., Pham, H.T.K., Neff, W., Nguyen, V.C., Tran, N.D., Kohei, T., Raymond, H., Kimberley, F. and Nguyen, T.H. (2015). Thirty years of vaccination in Vietnam: Impact and cost-effectiveness of the national expanded programme on immunization. Vaccine 33: 233–239.

[18] Morales, S.A., Kones, R. and Che, G.E. (2018). Barriers to global action plan for the prevention and control of non- communicable diseases: proposal modifications to the voluntary targets. *J Prev Med* 3: 1–5.

[19] Ngo, T.A. *et al.,* Improving technological process to produce hepatitis B DNA recombinant vaccine. State Pilot Production Project coded KC-10-06. Department of science and technology information, Hanoi, Vietnam.

[20] Nguyen T.V. *et al.,* Research on establishment of a Master Seed Virus System to use for production of anti-cervical cancer HPV vaccine. Independent State Research Subject coded 10/2012/HĐ-ĐTĐ, The Department of Science and Technology Information, Hanoi, Vietnam.

[21] Nguyen, T.V. *et al.,* Establish a technological process for manufacturing conjugate *Haemophilus influenzae* type b vaccine (Hib) in laboratory scale. State Research Subject coded KC.10.19/06-10, Department of science and technology information, Hanoi, Vietnam SDK: 2011-64-306 TTTTKHCNQG_8504.

[22] Nguyen, T.V. *et al.,* Establish a technological process for manufacturing influenza A/H5N1 in the laboratory scale. State Research Subject coded - DTDL 2006/02G, The Department of Information Science and Technology. SDK: 2007-64-109/KQNCTTTTKHCNQG_6374.

[23] Nguyen, T.V. *et al.,* Improving technological process for manufacturing the inactivated hepatitis A vaccine at the scale of 100,000 doses/year. State Research Subject codedKC-10-12. Department of science and technology information, Hanoi, Vietnam SDK: 2006-64-312 TTTTKHCNQG_5971.

[24] Nguyen, T.V. *et al.,* Improving technological process for manufacturing the inactivated hepatitis A vaccine at the scale of 100,000 doses/year. State Research Subject codedKC-10-12, Department of science and technology information, Hanoi, Vietnam SDK: 2006-64-312 TTTTKHCNQG_5971.

[25] Nguyen, T.V. *et al.,* State Research Subject coded KHCN-11-10: Study to receive technological transfers to build the production process for Hepatitis A and Hepatitis B DNA recombinant vaccines. Department of science and technology information, Hanoi, Vietnam.

[26] Nguyen, T.V. *et al.,* Technology and efficacy of the Micro-Elisa HBs Ag diagnostic kit and human plasma derived hepatitis B vaccine produced in Vietnam. State Research Subject coded KY 01-05, Department of Science and Technology Information. SDK, 96: 64–221.

[27] Pagliusi, S., Leite, L.C.C., Datla, M., *et al.* (2013). Developing countries vaccine manufacturer's network: Doing good by making high-quality vaccines affordable for all. *Vaccines* 31: 176–183.

[28] Raw, I. and Higashi, H.G. (1984). Self-sufficiency and innovation in vaccine production and public health. *Estud Avancados* 22: 155–170.

[29] UNICEF (2009). National EPI Review Report Program. p.1–57 https://www.unicef.org/vietnam/EPI_NATIONAL_Review_Report_Vietnam_2009_Final.pdf

[30] United Nations (2016). UN Documents: Gathering a body of global agreements. Sustainable Development http://www.un-documents.net/k-001303.htm

Vaccine Production in Nigeria: Transition from First to Third Generation Vaccines Production

O.O. Nwankiti[1] and T. Irhabor[2]

[1]Viral Research Division, National Veterinary Research Institute Vom, Plateau State, Nigeria

[2]Medical Laboratory Science Council of Nigeria, Abuja Nigeria

[1]E-mail: obee_nwankiti@yahoo.com

ABSTRACT: Vaccine, development and production is a constantly evolving area of science that exploits current biotechnological procedures, skills and technologies. These constantly evolving technologies pose challenges for developing countries especially in their transfer/adoption and establishment. Most vaccines used in developing countries are developed and produced in developed countries using isolates taken from the former. In most developing countries where vaccine production seemingly exists, they employ the first generation vaccine technology with challenges ranging from inadequate skilled personnel's, poor funding to antiquated facilities. Nigeria has a functional veterinary vaccine production facility and a non-functional human vaccine facility. The challenges towards transiting from first generation vaccine production to the new generation vaccines production in Nigeria may seem insurmountable and embarking on a transition to a tall order. Looking to the challenges Nigeria is facing in vaccine development, some prompt action is needed by the Government agencies. The corrective measures must be taken to a wide spread public health awareness for vaccine acceptance, along with an capacity building efforts to upgrade the infra-structure development, creating an enabling business environment, generation of skilled human resources. All this can be achieved only with willful political interventions, which can enable the Nigeria to a credible self-reliance vaccine production country.

Keywords: Developing Country, Vaccine Research and Development, Vaccines, Public-Private partnership, Good Manufacturing Processes (GMP), Biosafety Containment.

1. INTRODUCTION

Modern trends in vaccine research, development and production are constantly evolving, exploiting cutting edge biotechnological procedures and skills. These advancements have had their associated challenges especially in the transfer and establishment of these technologies between developed and developing countries (BioPharm 2011). What may be termed state-of-the art vaccine production technology/facility today most likely will be obsolete in a few years. Vaccine production and acceptance, distribution and trade between North-South collaborating partners and donor agencies can encourage or hinder a developing country from becoming self-sustaining in vaccines production because of interests from both sides (particularly the side of those importing these vaccines). The end user's interest most times is not the main focus.

2. BRIEF HISTORY OF VACCINE PRODUCTION IN NIGERIA

2.1 Veterinary Vaccines

Vaccine production in Nigeria started as early as 1924 after the establishment of a Veterinary Department in Zaria in the West African protectorate in 1913 to conduct livestock census, disease surveys, and disease control. In 1924, the Department was moved to Vom, a location on the 'Bauchi Plateau' as a veterinary laboratory and in the same year, the first biological (anti-rinderpest serum) was produced to control the rinderpest outbreaks. To date, the establishment (now called ***National Veterinary Research Institute, NVRI***) produces over 8 viral and 8 bacterial veterinary vaccines using cultural techniques of whole organisms *via* egg based, cell culture and a cellular methods. These methods have addressed issues like length of production processes, difficulty in scaling up production, high demands, and intermittent contamination from animal resources and most important is the high production cost. Currently, research is ongoing to combine these organisms as multivalent vaccines but still as whole organism and not as subunit vaccines (first generation vaccine production system). For years NVRI has been trying to scale up their production of first generation bacterial vaccines by building a gigantic manufacturing plant to meet local and international demand but this dream is yet to be achieved due to paucity of funds.

2.2 Human Vaccines

Nigerian Government established the ***Federal Vaccine Production Laboratory (FVPL),*** Yaba, Lagos in 1940 for the production of Anti-rabies, small-pox and yellow fever vaccines (mostly first generation vaccines) for local consumption and export. The facility was later shut down due to the inability of the FVPL to cope with operational challenges attributed to paucity of funds. In June 2016, the Federal Government of Nigeria and May & Baker Pharmaceuticals went into a Joint Venture Agreement for the production of local vaccines through Bio-vaccines Nigeria Limited. Quoting Prof. O. Tomori (Chairman of the Board for Bio-vaccines Nigeria limited), "We are not the first vaccine manufacturers in the world. The vaccines we have been using, others have been manufacturing it. So we are going to be working in partnership with people who are already producing vaccines. So our partnership includes getting some of what they are producing and finishing it up in Nigeria, making it a finished product, before we move on to producing our own vaccines" (Martins, 2018). This is termed a *'fill and finish'* method in vaccine manufacturing. This can be interpreted to mean that the proposed manufacture of vaccines is more of an assembly plant for vaccines using semi-finished products, not necessarily the development of new vaccines to meet demands for neither emerging and re-emerging diseases nor current trends in vaccine production since no facility upgrade from first generation vaccine production to current production trends were mentioned.

3. CURRENT TRENDS IN VACCINE PRODUCTION

Modern and emerging trends in vaccine development are focused on modular approach and multi-product, high end containment facilities (Wassard and Schubert 2012). With the use of genetic engineering and application of other state-of-the-art technologies for faster production *i.e.* single use technologies, reduction in logistics with focus on the certifiable product and its ease of reach to the end user, are the core competencies needs for effective production of new generation vaccines. Apart from those high end skills, there are several ground level competencies are also required towards vaccines of lower risks, which can easily developed from indigenous isolates, should be stable, lower production, handling and storage costs.

There are still several challenges surrounding the local production of first generation vaccines, keeping that in mind, will it be easy to migrate to production of third generation vaccines? There are plenty of questions that need to be asked like:

- Do we have enough infrastructures for vaccine development and production that can support the third generation vaccine production.
- Where from we will manage a high bio-safety containment facility for strain management.
- Do we have enough skilled human resources to develop a vaccine.
- Compliance with the international regulatory norms for certified vaccine production.

4. CHALLENGES IN THE PRODUCTION OF FIRST GENERATION VACCINES IN NIGERIA: TRANSITION TO CURRENT TREND OF VACCINE PRODUCTION

4.1 Research and Development

Research for vaccine development has not received the adequate attention and funding what it deserves. Pathogens responsible for diseases indigenous to Nigeria have been isolated but development as vaccine seed candidates have not been aggressively followed up hence vaccine seeds in current use are old isolates developed many years ago. There is currently no certified Type Culture Center in Nigeria for confirmation and storage of such vaccine seed candidates (from indigenous isolates), neither is there a certified vaccine seed bank. Most vaccine seeds used in today's production (even were locally isolated) were developed into vaccine seeds outside the country.

4.2 Technical/Skilled Human Resource Issues

Researchers in Nigeria are still grappling with the use of cell culture techniques and development of subunit vaccine candidates, hence the delay in migrating to second generation vaccines production. DNA technology which is the current trend in research is not routinely practiced in Nigeria. Molecular characterization of field isolates *via* sequencing is not routinely undertaken in Nigeria. Use of DNA vaccines is entirely foreign to Nigerians. There are no training facilities in Nigeria for vaccine technology. Most producers get on-the-job training. Training and retraining for skills acquisition towards research, development and manufacture of third generation vaccines is a prerequisite for vaccine production and transition to current trends.

4.3 Facility Set-ups

Facilities for modern production of vaccines focuses on containment systems at various bio-safety levels, facilities that meet ***Good Manufacturing Processes (GMP)***, easy and follow through quality control systems, manufacturing flexibilities, adaptability to change as demand, investment cost friendly for ease of even break, which is not in place yet. Modern facilities for research, development and manufacture of third generation vaccines will have to be setup and a gradual shift from production of first to third generation vaccines will be undertaken gradually. In many cases, it may be difficult to upgrade already existing facilities as their design and equipment's have become obsolete and do not meet modern day setups for current vaccine production trends, in this case it would be required to made investment in building new facility fulfilling core competencies of a modern facility.

4.4 Funding

Partnerships like that mentioned above between Government, May & Baker Pharmaceuticals and Bio-vaccines Nigeria limited with external funding will be needed to drive the setup of current vaccine production methods in Nigeria. Until funding agencies and investors see the need *via* a conducive and enabling business environment, they may be hesitate to be partner with exiting or prospective vaccine developers. As we need huge funds for vaccine research, development and production, we need to develop a framework for public-private partnership with potential business industries in vaccine development and promote private investment in this potential area.

4.5 Regulatory Agencies and Compliances

Vaccine development and production is a highly regulated activity and any installation involved in vaccine development and production should need to be adhered with the regulations laid by the international regulatory bodies for production of certified vaccines. Any produced vaccines need to be certified and regulated by an authorized body both with the national territory as well as by the international bodies. Veterinary vaccines produced in Nigeria are regulated by an authorized government approved agency Pan-African Veterinary Vaccines Center (PANVAC), situated in Ethiopia. Samples of produced batches of vaccines are sent for external quality control to PANVAC in Ethiopia and get certified. However, human vaccines that are produced in Nigeria were also need to compliance with the regulatory guidelines of WHO as it is applicable for the rest countries of the world. However, internal quality control measures at national level is needed to be devised by the Nigerian government to undertake full quality checks on every vaccine produced.

5. CONCLUSIONS

The challenges towards transiting from first generation vaccines production to current trends in vaccines production in Nigeria may seem insurmountable and embarking on a transition. If the following can be put in place: political and private sector will towards vaccine research, development and production, personnel and progressive infrastructure development, creation of an enabling business environment, wide spread public health awareness for vaccine acceptance and follow through regulations, the transition is achievable.

REFERENCES

[1] BioPharm International (2011). Challenges and trends in vaccine manufacturing. An evaluation of the technologies and process parameters needed to develop a safe, effective, and economically efficient vaccine. BioPharm International, Issue 7 http://www.biopharminternational.com/challenges-and-trends-vaccine-manufacturing

[2] Martins, I. (2018). Nigeria's Vaccine Production to be ready by 2021 - by Chairman, Board of Directors, Biovaccines Nigeria Limited, Prof. Oyewale Tomori. https://www.thisdaylive.com/index.php/2018/03/29/tomori-nigerias-vaccine-production-to-be-ready-by-2021

[3] NVRI (2018). History of the National Veterinary Research Institute Vom, Plateau State, Nigeria. www.nvri.gov.ng

[4] Wassard, K.H. and Schubert, H. (2012). Trends and challenges in large scale vaccines production in high containment environment. *55th ABSA Conference Orlando Florida.*

The Production and Use of Cell Culture Rabies Vaccine in Nepal

Bol Raj Acharya

Department of Livestock Services, Ministry of Agriculture, Land Management and Co-operatives, and Rabies Vaccine Production Laboratory, Veterinary Complex, Tripureshwor, Kathmandu, Nepal

E-mail: bolraj_acharya@yahoo.com, rbpl@gmail.com

ABSTRACT: Vaccination and adoption of proper bio security measures are the major ways to minimize the impact of disease problems. Rabies is fatal viral zoonoses transmitted from the rabid animals to other animals and to humans through their infected saliva (i.e. bites, scratches, licks on broken skin and mucous membrane). There is an estimated 55,000 human rabies related death worldwide every year of which, most cases occur in Asia and Africa with about 30,000 deaths in South Asia only. In Nepal, rabies is an important zoonotic disease that is taking lives of 100–200 human and around 350 animals every year. NeJaRab vaccine is an inactivated anti-rabies vaccine produced by infecting the BSR cells with PV/RV strains of rabies seed virus (developed from BHK 21, C13 cells from Pasteur Paris Institute) and inactivated with Beta Propiolactone (BPL). It is for veterinary use only and can be administered subcutaneous (SC) or intramuscular (IM). The vaccines undergo different tests required as per international standard like potency test, virus titration test, sterility test, staining test, inactivation test, stability test, toxicity test and safety test. The TCID50 is calculated and from which potency of the vaccine is finally determined. Similarly, LD50 is also determined form the back titration. The safety test is performed in unvaccinated dogs. The virus titer of this cell culture rabies vaccine is 2.5 IU which is in line with the standard of OIE (Office International des Epizooties i.e. World Organisation for Animal Health). Production of Cell Culture Rabies Vaccine for human use has been discontinued due to lack of resources and manpower.

Keywords: Nejarab, BPL, B.S.R. Cells, Rabies, TCID50, LD50, Toxicity and Safety Test.

1. INTRODUCTION

Nepal is one of the most resourceful countries in the world in terms of biodiversity due to its unique geographical and altitudinal location.

The elevation ranges from 60 m above sea level to the highest point on the earth, Mount Everest at 8,848 m, all within a distance of 150-kilometer resulting into climatic condition from subtropical to arctic. Nepal is a land locked country situated between 26°22′ to 30°27′ North latitudes and 80°4′ to 88°12′ East longitudes that covers a total land area of 147,181 sq. km.

Livestock makes a substantial contribution to household livelihoods of rural poor people, where poverty level is extremely high and more than 80% of the population relies on the agriculture. Diseases of livestock are the major problem in animal production as Nepal is endemic to many diseases of livestock which are responsible for huge economic losses (MOAD 2013). Besides this, prevalence of zoonotic diseases is also very high and pose constant threats to animals and human beings, rabies is among one of them. Rabies is fatal viral zoonoses transmitted from the rabid animals to other animals and to humans through their infected saliva (*i.e.* bites, scratches, licks on broken skin and mucous membrane). There is an estimated 55,000 human rabies related death worldwide every year of which, most cases occur in Asia and Africa with about 30,000 deaths in South Asia only (WHO, 2010). In Nepal, rabies is a dreaded zoonotic disease that takes 100–200 human lives and around 350 animals every year. The history of vaccine production in the country dates back to 1960, when a veterinary investigation laboratory was established in Kathmandu where the production of goat tissue vaccine for rinderpest was started (Singh 1990). Gradually, the production of other vaccines also began. Presently, the ***Central Biological Production Laboratory (CBPL)***, a fully government owned institute located in Kathmandu has been producing vaccines for a number of livestock diseases and the ***Rabies Vaccine Production Laboratory (RVPL)*** for rabies vaccine. The quantity of vaccine produced is very nominal when compared to national demand except for PPR and Swine Fever disease. In Nepal, the production of vaccines is mainly the business of government as the market is very small with minimum scope for exportation (Devleesschauwer *et al.*, 2016).

In Nepal, anti-rabies vaccine production was started from sheep brain (20 and 5% phenolized sheep brain) for the first time by the then Veterinary Laboratory in 1970, then in 1981, a separate laboratory ***Rabies Vaccine Production Laboratory (RVPL)*** was established for the production of rabies vaccine. Supply of the beta-propiolactone (BPL) inactivated Nerve Tissue Rabies Vaccine (NTV) for human use began in June 1986 after being certified by World Health Organization (WHO) and it was in use until December 30, 2006 (Devleesschauwer *et al.*, 2016), later WHO recommended a ban on the production of NTV because of its side effects. The cell culture rabies vaccine which was under research and development since 2002 was first commercial vaccine for the use on animal released in June 2006 with the technical support of Japan International Cooperation Agency (JICA), therefore, the vaccine was named NeJaRab (Pant 2013). Consecutive batches of vaccine were produced in the following years and tested through OIE (Office International des Epizooties i.e. World Organisation for Animal Health) Reference Laboratory, Agence Française de Sécurité Sanitaire des Aliments (AFSSA, Nancy Laboratory for Rabies and Wildlife), France in 2005. At present RVPL produces about 50,000 doses of cell culture rabies vaccine which is planning to scale up to 200,000 doses annually (Pant 2013, Devleesschauwer *et al.*, 2016). NeJaRab vaccine is an inactivated anti-rabies vaccine produced by infecting the BSR cells with PV/RV strain of rabies seed virus (developed from BHK 21, C13 cells in InstitutePasteur) and inactivated with Beta Propiolactone (BPL). It is for veterinary use only and can be administered intramuscular (IM), and/or subcutaneous (SC). Trial production of Cell Culture Rabies Vaccine for human use has been discontinued due to lack of separate laboratory facility and manpower.

2. MATERIALS AND METHODS

2.1 Production of Vaccine

Rabies vaccine production is performed in roller bottle since this method is easier and suitable for small scale production. The vaccine is produced using BHK-BSR cell line cultured in Minimum Essential Medium (MEM) with L-glutamine, antibiotics, antifungal and supplemented with 5% fetal bovine serum. For this vaccine, the PV/RV rabies virus strain vaccine seed is used. After restoration, the cell lines are multiplied initially in cell culture flasks then in roller bottles and the multiplication is continued until the required quantity of cells are achieved for one batch of production. The cells are then infected with the virus at the rate of 0.001/cell and incubated for 6 days at 37°C in roller apparatus. The bottles are placed horizontally on roller apparatus and rotated at a rate of 0.25 rpm at 37°C for 24 hours allowing infected cells to attach to the bottle surface, and then at 0.5 rpm for rest of the period. After the attachment of the infected cells to the bottle surface, the growth medium is replaced by a maintenance medium without serum. After 6 days of incubation, the vaccine is harvested and inactivated with ß-propiolactone then purified by centrifuging in continuous flow rotor (at 10,000 rpm). The rate of dilution of the β-propiolactone is 1/1000. The vaccine now is stored at 4°C for one week with shaking of bottle daily to facilitate proper mixing of β-propiolactone.

2.2 Quality Control Tests

The vaccines undergo different tests required as per international standard like potency, virus titration, sterility, staining, inactivation, stability, toxicity, specificity and safety test. It is mandatory that the vaccine to must pass all the control tests before it is released to the market. The vaccine has met the requirements of the World Organization for Animal Health (OIE) and World Health Organization (WHO).

2.3 Potency Test

Each batch of vaccine is passed through the NIH test for the rabies vaccine potency (Barth and Jaeger 1979). The potency of at least 1.0 International Unit (IU) per dose of vaccine is mandatory, which is acceptable as par international norms. The test measures the degree of protection conferred by inactivated rabies vaccines in vaccinated mice challenged with rabies virus. The test is conducted by vaccinating two groups of mice (4–5 weeks old), at 7 days and 14 days with dilution of a reference vaccine and the vaccine under test. 14 days after the last vaccination, the vaccinated mice and a control group of mice are challenged with the virus mouse-brain strain of fixed RV (rabies virus). The mice are observed for 14 days and the median Effective Dose (DE_{50}) of the reference and test vaccines is determined, based on the number of survivors. The relative potency of the test vaccine is then calculated by comparing the DE_{50} of the test vaccine with that of the reference vaccine. The virus titer of this cell culture rabies vaccine is more than 2.5 IU which is in line with the standard of OIE and WHO.

2.4 Neutralization Test

Since the facility in the laboratory for neutralization test does not exist, the serum samples from vaccinated dogs are sent to reference laboratories abroad. The results of the test indicate that the vaccine produces protective antibody level.

2.5 Filling into Bottles

After passing all the quality control tests the vaccine is to be filled into the bottles, with two different capacity levels: multi doses (10 ml) and single dose (1 ml) in a sterile environment.

2.6 Distribution

The multi dose bottles are handed over to the Department of Livestock Services free of cost to be used in vaccination camps and for post exposure prophylaxis especially in large animals. Single dose bottles are sold to the private practitioners through official dealers.

3. RESULTS AND DISCUSSION

The inactivated cell-culture rabies vaccine produced by RVPL has shown to be safe and highly effective, and fulfill the highest international standards set by the WHO and OIE. Cell culture technology is very much sensitive in terms of contamination from bacteria and fungi, therefore, a strict bio-containment measures has been adopted in the laboratory. It is essential to produce safe and potent vaccine, that we have a perfect cell-culture environment in the laboratory along with a GLP accredited bio-containment facility, in addition to a standard production protocol. The annual national demand of the veterinary rabies vaccine in the country is estimated to be 1 to 1.5 million doses, while internal production of the vaccine is about 50,000 doses and remaining vaccines are imported from outside. In recent years, the government has increased allocation of budget to upgrade the production capacity of the laboratory especially on infra-structure (BSL standard) and equipments in order to increase the production of the vaccine to meet the national demand. It is expected that in a couple of years the laboratory will be able to meet that target. In addition to this, with the improvement in the laboratory facility and increased resources the laboratory will be able to continue the production of rabies vaccine for human use as well.

REFERENCES

[1] Ahmad, Fayaz, Zaverrie, A., Howaizi, N. and Eslami, N.; Production of Rabies Vaccine Using BHK-21 with Roller Bottle Cell Culture Technique. Iranian Biomedical Journal, 1 (1): 35–38 (1997).

[2] Annual Technical Report (2016/17), Directorate of Animal Health, Department of Livestock Services, Government of Nepal, Tripureshwor, Kathmandu, Nepal.

[3] Barth, R. and Jaeger, O. (1979). NIH potency tests with inactivated rabies vaccines. *Zentralbl Bakteriol B* 169: 488–94.

[4] Devleesschauwer, B., Aryal, A., Sharma, B.K., *et al.* (2016). Epidemiology, Impact and Control of Rabies in Nepal: A Systematic Review. *PLoS Negl Trop Dis* 10:e0004461. Published 2016 Feb. 12.

[5] MOAD (2013). Agriculture and livestock Insurance Policy, Ministry of Agricultural Development, Kathmandu (Nepal).

[6] OIE Manual of Diagnostic Tests and Vaccines (2013). Chapter 2.1.13., 2013. Office International Des Epizooties (OIE), Paris, France.

[7] Pant, G.R. (2013). Rabies Control Strategy in SAARC Member Countries. World Organisation of Animal Health (OIE), Kathmandu (Nepal).

[8] Singh, U. (1990). Current Situation of Rinderpest in Nepal. Ministry of Agriculture, Department of Livestock Services, Kathmandu (Nepal).

Field Trial of a Newcastle Disease I-2-6 Grain Adapted Pelleted Feed Vaccine (NDVI-2-6 GAPFV) in Five Selected Rural Communities in Nigeria

Anthony N. Egbuji[1], John O. Ibu[2], Ismali A. Shittu[1], Dauda G. Bwala[1], Anna S. Lohlum[1], Enurah L. Uwanibe[1], Josephine A. Kiagama[1], Evelyn D. Dung[1], Davou C. Nyam[1], Adamu C. Kwanga[1], Akachi U. Kenneth[1], Raymond C. Obene[1], Nicodemus M. Useh[2] and Jude S. Rabo[2]

[1]National Veterinary Research Institute, Vom, Plateau State, Nigeria

[2]University of Agriculture, Makurdi, Benue State, Nigeria

*E-mail: wisemenvet@yahoo.com

ABSTRACT: *Field trial of the NDVI-2-6 GAPFV was carried out in five selected rural communities of Jos South Local Government Area of Plateau state Nigeria to determine efficacy of the NDVI-2-6 GAPFV in eliciting production of protective detectable Newcastle disease (ND) antibodies in selected unvaccinated rural scavenging chickens under field situation. In this study, a total of four hundred and eighty seven (487) rural scavenging chickens were selected, tagged and vaccinated with the NDVI-2-6 GAPFV. Serum samples were collected and tested pre- and post-vaccination. The samples were analyzed using the haemagglutination (HA) and haemagglutination inhibition (HI) assays. The result of the pre-vaccination study showed complete absence of ND antibodies in the unvaccinated chickens with mean HI titre of* $\leq 2\ log_2$ *while sequel to the administration of NDVI-2-6 GAPFV to the selected unvaccinated chickens HI of* $\geq 2\ log_2$ *was recorded. The geometric mean titer (GMT) range of 9.2 to 36.1 was recorded four weeks post vaccination. The statistical analysis of the study revealed that the NDVI-2-6 GAPFV was able to elicit production of protective antibodies in the vaccinated flock at a p value of < 0.001. The result of this study also revealed presence of detectable antibodies twelve weeks post-vaccination, with evidence of antibody weaning observed.*

Keywords: Newcastle Disease Pelleted Feed Vaccine, Rural Scavenging Chickens.

1. INTRODUCTION

Newcastle disease (ND) is a highly contagious viral disease affecting wild and domestic avian species (Seal *et al.,* 2000, Aldous *et al.,* 2003). The impact of ND is most notable in domestic poultry due to their high susceptibility and the severe consequences of virulent ND strains outbreaks in this flock (Alexander 1988a, 2001, Alders and Spradbrow 2001b). Since, ND was first reported in Nigeria in 1953 at Ibadan (Hill *et al.,* 1953), it has become the most important viral disease of chicken and widely spread throughout the country with annual epidemics being recorded in highly susceptible poultry flocks (Aliyu *et al.,* 2015). The high genetic diversity of the virus could have contributed to the increasing rate of the disease (Aliyu *et al.,* 2015). In Nigeria ND is generally well-recognized by farmers in both local and exotic breed (Lawal *et al.,* 2015). The NDVI-2 vaccine was discovered after an extensive screening of NDV isolates by scientists at the University of Queensland in Australia (Spadbrow *et al.,* 1995, Bensink and Spradbrow 1999) and the vaccine strain has been extensively tested to protect rural poultry in Asia and Africa (Tu *et al.,* 1998, Wambura *et al.,* 2000, Wambura *et al.,* 2007). The search for a suitable food material as vaccine carrier has however, been attempted in several countries with limited successes (Spradbrow 1987).

Most of the investigations of food carriers for thermo stable ND vaccine have been undertaken in Asia, Africa, and Australia (Spradbrow 1992, Ibrahim *et al.,* 1992, Wambura *et al.,* 2007). In Asia, suitable food carriers used include paddy (unhusked) rice, cooked white rice and cooked parboiled rice. Uncooked white rice is not a suitable food carrier. For most grains 7–10 g per chicken is recommended. For cooked white rice 20 g is required for each chicken (Spradbrow 2002). There have been fewer studies on foodstuffs, especially the available grains in Africa. In Ethiopia, parboiled barley was shown to be a suitable carrier for NDVI-2 vaccine. Here we used *Digitalia iburua* as a vaccine virus carrier and the obtained results are discussed.

2. MATERIALS AND METHODS

2.1 Materials

Pelleted ND feed vaccine was produced using heat treated *Digitalia iburua* and a heat modified wet NDVI-2-6 (Egbuji *et al.,* 2017). The EID_{50} of the grain adapted (NDVI-2-6 GAPFV) vaccine was determine in chicken embryonated eggs and calculated using the Spearman-Kaaber formula. The calculated EID_{50} was within the expected dose range for

NDVI-2 standard vaccine. The feed vaccine was administered to the selected flock at a dose of 20 g per bird. Vaccinated birds were tagged and blood sample were collected for serum harvest fortnightly for detection of presence of anti-NDVI-2-6 GAPFV antibodies.

2.2 Blood Samples

Blood samples were aseptically collected from the wing vein of selected flock; usually 0.5 to 1.0 ml per bird with using sterile disposable syringes. Samples were allowed to clot in syringes and left overnight at room temperature for complete serum separation. The separated serum was harvested and consequently frozen at –20°C this was later used for haemagglutination inhibition (HI) test.

2.3 Haemagglutination and Haemagglutination Inhibition

A 1% suspension of chicken red blood cells (RBCs) was prepared for use in haemagglutination (HA) and haemagglutination inhibition (HI) tests according to (OIE 2010). The HA titres of standard NDV antigen was determined as described by Allan and Gough (1974) and diluted to contain 4 HA units. The reconstituted antigen containing the 4 HA units was used in the determination of test sera titers in the HI test. The HI titer for each screened serum was determined and expressed in log_2, and the geometric mean titer was calculated for each sampled village. Any HI titer $\geq 2\ log_2$ was considered positive.

3. RESULT

The results in Table 1 showed that anti-ND antibody was completely absent in all the screened sera collected before vaccination from the studied five villages.

Table 1: Result of the HI assay on sera collected from pre-vaccinated free range domestic chickens from *Du*, *Ngohong*, *Chaha*, *Chakarum* and *Chele* in Jos South local government area of Plateau State

Villages	*Number of Birds Screened*	*Vaccination Record/History*	*Mean HI Titres*
Chaha	130	Nil	$\leq 2\ \log_2$
Ngohong	72	Nil	$\leq 2\ \log_2$
Du	57	Nil	$\leq 2\ \log_2$
Chakarum	155	Nil	$\leq 2\ \log_2$
Chele	73	Nil	$\leq 2\ \log_2$
Total	487	Nil	GMT 0

Results in Table 2 showed detected anti-ND antibody in each of the vaccinated flock at week 1, 2, 4, and 12 post vaccination and their various ***Geometric Mean Titers (GMT).***

Table 2: Sero-prevalence of Newcastle Diseases antibody in free range domesticated chickens in *Du, Ngohong, Chaha, Chakarum* and *Chele* villages in Jos south local government area Plateau state at different time points post vaccination

Villages	*Number of Birds Screened*	*Week-1*	*Week-2*	*Week-4*	*Week-12*
		Anti-body titre/GMT			
		Prevac	*Postvac*	*Postvac*	*Postvac*
Chaha	130	$\leq 2\ log_2$; GMT = 0	16.0	18.0	8.0
Ngohong	72	$\leq 2\ log_2$; GMT = 0	9.2	21.1	12.0
Du	57	$\leq 2\ log_2$; GMT = 0	8.6	19.7	11.0
Chakarum	155	$\leq 2\ log_2$; GMT = 0	11.0	24.5	13.0
Chele	73	$\leq 2\ log_2$; GMT = 0	12.0	36.1	18.0

Geometric Mean Antibody Titre (GMT)

Table 3 shows the statistical analysis of post-vaccination results for birds in the five studied villages. In *Du* village, the mean value was significantly ($p < 0.05$) higher at week-4 post vaccination than at week-2 post-vaccination. Similar results were obtained in vaccinated poultry from *Chaha* and *Ngo Hong*. The detectable antibodies peaked at week-4 in the screened localities by the 12th week and, an evidence of antibody weaning was observed.

Table 3: Result of Post-vaccination Sero-monitoring for Birds in the Field Trial

Villages	*Vaccination Period*	*Mean ± SD*	*F-test*	*P*
Du	Pre vaccination 2 weeks post vaccination 4 weeks post vaccination	1.0 ± 0.0^a 2.4 ± 0.9^b 3.2 ± 0.5^c	392.466	0.001
Chaha	Pre vaccination 2 weeks post vaccination 4 weeks post vaccination	1.0 ± 0.0^a 2.3 ± 0.5^b 3.2 ± 0.6^c	473.147	0.001
Ngo Hong	Pre vaccination 2 weeks post vaccination 4 weeks post vaccination	1.0 ± 0.0^a 2.4 ± 0.5^b 3.2 ± 0.6^c	787.195	0.001
Chakarum	Pre vaccination 3 weeks post vaccination 3 months post vaccination	1.0 ± 0.2^a 4.8 ± 1.5^b 5.2 ± 1.8^c	440.774	0.001
Chele	Pre vaccination 3 weeks post vaccination 3 months post vaccination	1.4 ± 0.5^a 4.9 ± 1.9^b 4.3 ± 1.0^c	153.460	0.001

Row with different superscripts is statistically significantly different at $p < 0.001$.

4. DISCUSSIONS

Pre-vaccination screening of the selected flock showed that all the screened birds lack anti-NDV antibodies. This result was in agreement with the flock history, as none of the sampled birds had history of ND vaccination. This could probably explain the usually high morbidity and mortality amongst this flock during the occasional Newcastle disease outbreak. Based on the pre-vaccination results, birds were given NDVI-2-6 GAPFV at a dose of 20 g per chicken. The vaccinated flocks were sampled at Weeks 1, 2, 4 and 12 respectively. The obtained results revealed a steady increase in the GMT post-vaccination, with titers increasing from $\leq 2\ log_2$ pre-vaccination to $\geq 2\ log_2$ post-vaccination. This suggests sero-conversion sequel to feed vaccine administration. These results show that pelleted NDVI-2-6 GAPFV was able to elicit production of detectable anti-NDV antibodies in vaccinated flocks under field situation. The P value of ($p < 0.001$) showed that the post-vaccination results were significantly higher than pre-vaccination ones, thus, NDVI-2-6 GAPFV may confer protection in the event of wild viral ND challenge. The application of the NDVI-2-6 GAPFV will minimize the stress associated with flock vaccination especially in rural setting since handling of individual birds for vaccination purposes will be minimal and the technicality of vaccine administration will be eliminated by feed-based vaccines as minimal expertise will be required for its administration.

Evidence of antibodies weaning was observed on Week-12 post-vaccination (see Table 2) suggesting the need for a booster vaccination at this stage. This is similar to the findings of Wambura *et al.,* (2000) where protective ND antibodies where still detectable 90 days post administration of NDVI-2 vaccine to commercial and rural backyard birds in Tanzania. It was equally suggested by Abdi *et al.* (2016) that repeated vaccination induces progressively higher HI antibody titers that could correspond to high levels of protection.

Nigeria has an estimated poultry population of 140 million with backyard poultry production accounting for more than 60% of the total flock with an asset value of > 5.75 billion US Dollars (Nnadi *et al.,* 2010). However, annual loss due to seasonal outbreak of ND discourages the rural dwellers from investing in rural backyard poultry farming, despite its derivable economic benefits. Vaccination against Newcastle Disease has been reported as the major safe guard against ND outbreaks especially in countries with endemic very virulent Newcastle Disease (*vv*ND) and highly deficient biosafety control measures (Allan *et al.*, 1978, Aini *et al.*, 1990 and Usman 2002).

Though numerous ND vaccines abounds, their use in rural backyard poultry production are often limited and of minimal effect unlike what is obtainable in commercial poultry production, where effective utilization of ND vaccine is routinely applied to control the Newcastle disease outbreaks. Therefore, a mandatory strategic vaccination of rural poultry flock will mitigate against seasonal outbreaks of ND in these flock (Egbuji *et al.*, 2017a). Though, ND can be controlled by flock vaccination. This is rarely carried out on rural backyard poultry flock due to lack of awareness on the part of the flock owners, knowledge of the available vaccine and their application. Current ND vaccines which are available come in large dose units and are targeted towards large commercial flocks. These vaccines have little relevance in village backyard poultry flocks which are often small, scattered, multi-aged, and free-roaming with minimal control. Maintenance of cold chain for vaccine viability is also difficult in rural setting due unavailability of electricity for vaccine storage. These challenges can be managed by development of heat resistant grain adapted pelleted feed vaccine, for rural backyard poultry protection against ND outbreak.

The consequences of ND outbreaks are more in Nigeria where over 60% of the poultry population are rural, that are left to roam freely to scavenge for food and water thus, bringing them in close contact with wild birds (Adene and Oguntade 2006), that might harbor wild virulent ND virus. Therefore, the establishment of a strategic vaccination programme using NDVI-2-6 GAFPV geared towards eradication of ND especially in rural backyard poultry flock cannot be overemphasized. We believed that NDVI-2-6 GAFPV can contribute in no small measures to solving ND challenge in rural backyard poultry flocks, since the vaccine will easily be administered and stress associated with handling of individual birds, and water deprivation will be eliminated by the application of feed-based vaccine. The introduction of NDVI-2-6 GAFPV will enable rural poultry farmers; take charge of ND outbreak in their flock as little expertise will be required in the administration of the pelleted feed vaccine.

5. CONCLUSION AND SUGGESTIONS

Our results suggest that scavenging birds in the sampled communities were all vulnerable to wild ND virus outbreak; this might explain the occasionally high morbidity and mortality rate recorded during ND outbreaks. The findings of our study reveal that adoption of NDVI-2-6 GAFPV as an alternative to conventional ND vaccine in rural settings.

ACKNOWLEDGEMENTS

We are sincerely grateful to the Competitive Agricultural Research Scheme (CARGS) under Agriculture Research Council of Nigeria (ARCN) for providing funds for this research work and the National Veterinary Research Institute, Vom for providing the enabling environment for this research project.

REFERENCES

[1] Adene, D.F. and Oguntade, A.E. (2006). The structural and importance of commercial and rural based poultry industry in Nigeria. *Nigerian Poultry Sector Report* FAO, Rome, pp. 1–70.

[2] Alders, R.G. and Spradbrow, P.B. (2001b). SADC *Planning Workshop on Newcastle Disease Control in Village Chickens.* Proceedings of an International Workshop, Maputo, Mozambique, 6–9 March 2000. *ACIAR Proceedings* 103, 158pp.

[3] Aldous, E.W., Mynn, J.K. and Alexander, D.J. (2003). A molecular epidemiology study of avian paramyxovirus type 1 (Newcastle disease) isolate by phylogenetic analysis of a partial nucleotide sequence of the fusion protein gene. *Avian Pathology* 32: 239–256.

[4] Alexander, D.J. (2001). Newcastle disease—The Gordon Memorial Lecture. *British Poultry Science,* 42: 5–22.

[5] Alexander, D.J. (1988a). Preface: In: *Newcastle Disease,* D.J. Alexander, Ed., Kluwer Academic Publishers, Boston, p. XI.

[6] Aliyu, H.B., Saidu, L., Abdu, P.A. and Oladele, S.B. (2015). A retrospective analysis of Newcastle disease diagnosed at poultry clinic of Ahmadu Bello University, Zaria, Nigeria. *Sokoto Journal of Veterinary Sciences,* 13: 42–48.

[7] Allan, W.H. and Gough, E. (1974). A standard haemagglutination inhibition test for Newcastle disease a comparison of macro and micro methods. *Vet Rec.,* 95: 120–123.

[8] Bensink Z. and Spradbrow P. 1999. Newcastle disease virus strain I-2—A prospective thermostable vaccine for use in developing countries. *Veterinary Microbiology* 68: 131–139

[9] Egbuji, A.N., John, O.I., Ismali, A.S., Echeonwu, G.O.N., Enura, L.U., Dauda, B., Josphine, K., Evelyn, D., Davou, N., Chinemerem, O., Adamu, K., Fatima, M., Haruna, D., Sati, L., Nicodemus, U. and Jude, R. (2017). Screening of rural scavenging birds for the presence of detectible protective Newcastle disease antibodies in some selected rural communities of Plateau State. *African Journal of Microbiology Research* 11: 1431–1433.

[10] Egbuji, N.A., John, O.I., Ismaila, A.S., Dauda, G.B., Anne, S.L., Josephine, K., Evelyn, D.D., Enurah, L.U., Fatima, B.M., Dung, S.L., Chinemerem, R.O., Choji, A.K., Nicodemus, M.U., Paul, A.A., Usman, M., John, A.O. and Jude, S.R. (2017b). Immune profiling of grain adapted I-2 (GAI-2) pelleted

feed vaccine in 6 weeks old cockerels in Vom Nigeria. *Journal of Experimental Biology and Agricultural Sciences,* 5: 599–605.

[11] Ibrahim, A.L., Ideris, A. and Babjee, A.M. (1992). An overview of the use of food-based Newcastle disease vaccine in Malaysia. In: Spradbrow, P.B., ed., *Proceedings of an international workshop, Kuala Lumpur, 6–10 October 1991* Canberra, *ACIAR proceedings,* No. 39, pp. 75–79.

[12] Lawal, J.R., Jajere, S.M., Mustapha, M., Bello, A.M., Wakil, Y., Geidam, Y.A., Ibrahim, U.I. and Gulani, I.A. (2015). Prevalence of Newcastle Disease in Gombe, Northeastern Nigeria: A ten-year retrospective study (2004–2013). *British Microbiology Research Journal,* 6: 367–375.

[13] Nnadi, P.A. and George, S.O. (2010). A cross sectional survey on parasites of chickens in selected villages in the sub humid zones of South-Eastern Nigeria. *Journal of Parasitology Research,* 4: 1–6.

[14] OIE (2010). Newcastle Disease—Manual of standard for diagnostic tests and vaccines. *Office International des Epizootics* (OIE), Paris, p. 221–232.

[15] Seal, B.S., King, D.J. and Sellers, H.S. (2000). The avian response to Newcastle disease virus. *Developmental and Comparative Immunology,* 24: 257–268.

[16] Spadbrow, P.B. and Sabine, M. (1995). Australian studies on Newcastle disease virus. *The French heritage Vet Microbiol,* 46: 11–12.

[17] Spradbrow, P. (1992). A review of the use of food carriers for the delivery of oral Newcastle disease vaccine. In: Spradbrow, P.B., ed., *Proceedings of an international workshop, Kuala Lumpur,* 6–10 October 1991. Canberra, *ACIAR proceedings,* No. 39, p. 18–20.

[18] Spradbrow, P.B. (1987). Newcastle disease in Australia. In: *Newcastle disease in poultry: a new food pellet vaccine. The Australian Centre for International Agricultural Research,* Canberra, pp. 40–43.

[19] Tu, T.D., Phuc, K.V., Dinh, N.T.K. Quoc, D.N and Spradbrow, P.B. (1998). Vietnamese trials with a thermostable Newcastle disease vaccine (strain I-2) in experimental and village chickens. *Preventive Veterinary Medicine,* 34: 205–214.

[20] Usman, M.U. (2002). Effects of vaccination of chickens against Newcastle diseases with thermostable V4 and La Sota vaccines. *MSc Thesis.* Department of Veterinary Surgery and Medicine, Ahmadu Bello University, Zaria, Nigeria.

[21] Wambura, P.N., Meers, J. and Spradbrow, P. (2007). Survival of avirulent thermostable Newcastle disease virus (strain I-2) in raw, baked, oiled, and cooked white rice at ambient temperatures. *J Vet Sci.,* 8: 303–308.

[22] Wambura, P.N., Kapaga, A.M. and Hyera, J.M.K. (2000). Experimental trials with thermostable Newcastle disease virus (strain I-2) in commercial and village chickens in Tanzania. *Preventive Veterinary Medicine,* 43: 75–83.

Water Transmitted Viruses in River Nile Basin Countries: Pathogenesis, Prevalence and Vaccine Availability

Dina Nadeem Abd-Elshafy[1, 2] **and Mahmoud Mohamed Bahgat**[2, 3]

[1]Environmental Virology Laboratory, Department of Water Pollution Research, Division of Environmental Research, the National Research Centre, Giza 12311, Egypt

[2]Research Group Immune- and Bio-markers for Infection, the Centre of Excellence for Advanced Science, the National Research Centre, Giza 12311, Egypt

[3]Department of Therapeutic Chemistry, Division of Pharmaceutical and Drug Industries Research, the National Research Centre, Dokki, Giza 12311, Egypt

E-mail: [1]dnanadeem@yahoo.com

ABSTRACT: The River Nile serves as the main source of drinking water to eleven (11) countries namely Tanzania, Uganda, Rwanda, Burundi, the Democratic Republic of the Congo, Kenya, Ethiopia, Eritrea, South Sudan, Sudan and Egypt. Water treartment plants are unsufficiently distributed among all the areas in these countries due to their poor economic status and as such it has been reported that the untreated sewage water is disposed into the River Nile thus, represents the main source of water contamination including the viruses. We aimed to collect all the reports showing the presence of all water-borne viruses in River Nile water of all those countries. Keywords used were combinations between name of virus and name of country or name of virus and pathogenesis or name of virus and vaccine availability. The search was made in Pubmed, WHO library, science direct and specialized medical websites collecting all the available data between 1988–2018. Many reports showed presence of nearly all known water-borne viruses in all the named eleven countries inclusive of the Nile water, sewage water and/or reticulated water. Further analysis indicated that some countries such as Egypt, Sudan and Kenya have already reported the presence of all known water-borne viruses. This does not mean absence of viruses in the rest of the eleven countries only it showed that reports containing information about these three countries are available and more reports are needed for the other countries. Obviously,vaccines are available for some of these water borne viruses namely;adenovirus, rotavirus, hepatitis A virus, hepatitis E virus and poliovirus, but no vaccines are available for astrovirus, norovirus, coxsackie A virus, coxsackie B virus and echovirus.

Keywords: Water-borne Viruses, Pathogenesis, Prevalence, Vaccines, River Nile Basin Countries.

1. INTRODUCTION

River Nile is the most important source of drinking water to many African countries but these countries play a major role in contaminating the river body and its tributatries. It is reported that indiscriminate dumping of refuse and sewage materials from the river Nile connected countries occur frequently (Rosenbaun, 1994). Therefore, all the sewage contaminants including bacteria, parasites and viruses can easily reach the River Nile through its tributaries making it the source of transmitting pathogenic organism to healthy people by drinking, showering or swimming through fecal-oral route or via the nose or eyes (Farthing, 1989).

This review shows the role of River Nile basin countries in contamination and spread of disease-causing viruses. Objective issues addressed by the group included:

1. Role of River Nile basin countries in the spread of water-borne viruses among their population.
2. Characteristics and pathogenesis of the transmitted viruses via the Nile water.
3. Prevalence of water-borne viruses in the eleven river Nile basin countries.
4. Vaccine availability against the disease causing viruses.

The eleven countries benefitting from the River Nile are: Tanzania, Uganda, Rwanda, Burundi, the Democratic Republic of the Congo, Kenya, Ethiopia, Eritrea, South Sudan, Sudan and Egypt (Oloo, 2007). Due to lack of appropriate water treatment plants and adequate pollution control implementation mechanism, untreated sewage water from the 11 countries is discharged into the said river thus, considered to be the main source of pollution and transmission of water-borne viruses (El-Sayed and Salem, 2005). Sewage water contains a number of microbial pollutants including viruses. According to the World Health Organization (WHO), a number of viruses are considered to cause water related infections, these include adenovirus, astrovirus, hepatitis A and E viruses, rotavirus, norovirus and enteroviruses such as coxsackie viruses and Polioviruses (Aimee, 2015). Reports showed the presence of most of these viruses in nearly all the River Nile basin countries. Some viruses were detected in the River Nile water, in sewage water while the majority is reported as infections among inhabiting human populations and references for this will be shown in result section.

These pathogenic organisms cause different types of diseases which may be transmitable in the human population such as pharyngitis, gastroenteritis, hepatitis and diarrhea which are most common among the children.

Notably, while vaccines are available for adenovirus, rotavirus, hepatitis A virus, hepatitis E virus and poliovirusto lower and eradicate prevalence of infections within the human population, no vaccines are available for astrovirus, norovirus, coxsackie A virus, coxsackie B virus and echovirus.

2. MATERIAL AND METHODS

A total of 150 references were used including the research articles, websites, book chapters and reviews. Keywords used were combinations between name of virus and name of country or name of virus and pathogenesis or name of virus and vaccine availability. The search was made in PubMed, WHO library, science direct and specialized medical websites collecting all the available data between 1988–2018.

3. RESULTS AND DISCUSSION

3.1 Evidence of Country-Specific Water Contamination of the River Nile Basin Countries

The River Nile can be contaminated with the human excreta either by land run-off or dumping of the sewage into river or lakes (Figure 1).

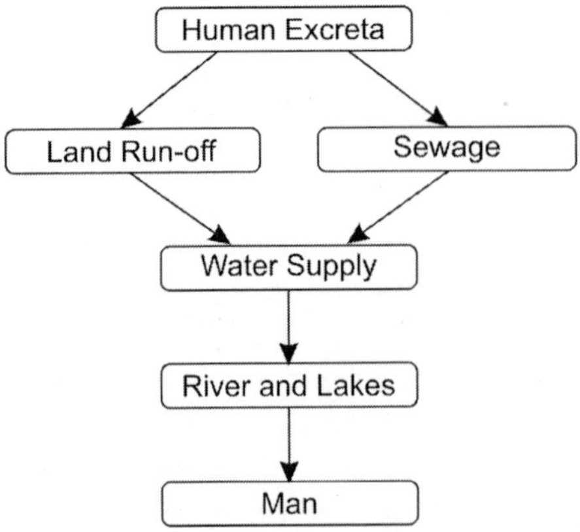

Fig. 1: Route of Water-borne Virus Transmission to Human (Rao and Melnick, 1986)

Egypt

Sewage water (Ecomina, 2017) as well as industrial waste (El-Sayed and Salem, 2005) from many areas in Egypt are discharged untreated into the river due to lack of water treatment plants and this are considered to be the main source of pollution to the Nile water (Abd El-Hady, 2014) from Aswan to Delta (Shamrukh and Abdel-Wahab, 2011).

It is expected that pollution level will increase specially after establishing the Ethiopian Dam, as a result, expected lowering of the Nile water level with the same number and levels of contaminants (Shamrukh and Abdel-Wahab, 2011; Ezzat *et al.*, 2012; Goher *et al.*, 2014), will mean that if 100 viral particles are recovered from 1 liter of Nile water, in case of lowering water level, it will be recovered from 800 ml.

Sudan

Although in 2004, the WHO estimated that improved drinking water quality has reached 70% of Sudan's population, the reality is that the access to water and sanitation is extremely low in rural areas which represent 42% of the Sudanese population. Around 12.9% of new born babies die as a result of diarrheal (USAID, 2006) caused by drinking the contaminated water.

Eritrea

Pollution monitored in 40–90% of water sources during the Rural Water Point National Inventory was found to contain biological contaminants (FAO, 2005).

Ethiopia

Fecal contaminants was reported in the water of River Nile (Goshu *et al.*, 2017) as well as in **Rwanda** (UNEP, 1999).

Lake Victoria was found to be polluted by discharge from the sewage effluent outlet that runs into it (Nilerak, 2005). It is the chief reservoir of the River Nile lying mainly in Tanzania and Uganda as well as on the borders of Kenya (Britannica, 2017).

Burundi

Water pollution is the main man-made source of pollution especially in rural areas as a result of sewage discharge (Nilerak, 2005).

3.2 Human Viruses in Water

Viruses are considered to be one of the important causes of water-related diseases. They might reach drinking water through contamination by human urine or feces of infected persons through sewage discharge (Farthing, 1989).

Viruses might reach uninfected person not only through contact or consumption of contaminated water but also via inhalation during showering, contact with skin and eyes during swimming (Aimee, 2015). Water-borne viruses can be classified into DNA and RNA viruses.

According to WHO, a number of viruses are considered to cause water-related infections. These include adenovirus, astrovirus, hepatitis A and E viruses, rotavirus, norovirus and enteroviruses [coxsackieviruses] and polioviruses (WHO, 2011).

3.2.1 *DNA Viruses*

(a) *Adenoviruses*

Classification and Characteristics

These are members of the family *Adenoviridae*. They are non-enveloped viruses with a double stranded DNA genome (Hogg, 2000; Thompson *et al.*, 2003).

Adenoviruses are stable to chemical or physical agents and different pH conditions that make them able to survive outside the body and water. Adenoviruses resist UV radiation (Thurston-Enriquez *et al.*, 2003; Wan and De Gregori, 2000). They spread via respiratory droplets and also by fecal-oral routes (Mickan and Kok, 1994) through contaminated water (Metzgar *et al.*, 2005).

Pathogenesis

Adenoviruses infect upper respiratory tract of humans and often cause conjunctivitis and tonsillitis, bronchiolitis or pneumonia especially in children. It can also cause viral meningitis or encephalitis. Infection with adenoviruses might also result in gastroenteritis. Self-recovery is the common end to adenovirus infection but this is not the case with immune deficient persons (Thacker *et al.*, 2009).

Prevalence in the River Nile Basin Countries

Different studies reported adenovirus but mainly in human samples. In Egypt a study showed that Adenovirus is common among patients having influenza like symptoms (Demian *et al.*, 2014). The same was shown from a study on human samples from northern Sharquiya and Demiatt, and southern, Menia and Aswan, Egyptian Governorates (Thacker *et al.*, 2009), with about 20% prevalence rates among children (Zaki and Abo El Kheir, 2017). Similarly, in Sudan 16.2% of patients suffering from diarrhea were found to be infected with adenovirus (Sudan *et al.*, 2013).

Human adenovirus was also reported in Kenya (Onyango and Angienda, 2010) and in Congo in 5% of children (Mayindou *et al.*, 2016).

Similar, infection reported in Uganda (Chen *et al.*, 2010) where in 65% of stool samples (Pauly *et al.*, 2014) and in Tanzania the virus was detected both in the diarrheic and non-diarrheic stool samples of children (Moyo *et al.*, 2014).

Conversly, no reports were found for adenovirus infection from Eritrea, Ethiopia, Ruanda and Burundi.

Vaccine Availability

Adenovirus vaccine is available. It contains both live adenovirus Type 4 and Type 7 and prevents illness caused by these two virus types. It is given in the form of tablets but as it is a living virus it is contraindicated to people under 17 or over 50 years as well as pregnant or lactating women.

It is recommended by the Department of Defense for military recruits entering basic training. It may also be recommended for other military personnel at high risk for adenovirus infection (CDC, 2014).

3.2.2 *RNA Viruses*

Double stranded RNA viruses

(a) *Rotavirus*

Classification and Characteristics: They belong to family *Reoviridae.* They are non-enveloped viruses with double stranded RNA genome (Bernstein, 2009). They are the most common cause of diarrheal among children (Dennehy, 2015). Every child in the world received rotavirus infection at least once by the age of five (Bernstein, 2009). About 37% of child death resulting from diarrhea is attributable to rotavirus (Tate *et al.*, 2016).

Pathogenesis: Rotavirus is transmitted by the fecal-oral route (Butz *et al.*, 1993) and possibly through the respiratory route (Dennehy, 2000). Rotavirus infection is accompanied by nausea, vomiting, watery diarrhea and low-grade fever. Once a child is infected by the virus, there is an incubation period of about two days before appearance of the symptoms (Hochwald and Kivela, 1999).

Post infection, vomiting is the first sign followed by diarrhoea, therefore, dehydration is common in rotavirus infection than infection by any other pathogen and represents the main cause of death (Hochwald and Kivela, 1999).

Prevalence in River Nile Basin Countries: The virus has been detected in human and environmental samples in many of the River Nile basin countries including Egypt where it was shown to infect 76.9% of Egyptian population having gastroenteritis and be the main causative agent of the disease in infants and children (Ibrahim, *et al.*, 2015; Ahmed *et al.*, 2014; Naficy *et al.*, 1999; Hashem *et al.*, 2012). Reports indicate that isolates have being confirmed from the samples collected from sewage (Villena *et al.*, 2003) and the Nile water (El-Senousy *et al.*, 2014).

In Sudan rotavirus infection was reported among under 5 years' children (Magzoub *et al.*, 2013), and around 84% of patients having viral diarrhea were found infected with rotavirus as a result of drinking untreated water (Demian, *et al.*, 2014). In Eritrea, rotavirus was found to be the cause of 28% of under-five diarrheal hospitalization (WHO, 2014a). Also it causes death of about 700 Eritrean children under 5 each year and considered the common cause of fatal diarrhea in young children worldwide (WHO, 2014b; Tate *et al.*, 2008).

The high prevalence rate made it important to be recommended for all those travelling to Eritrea to consider all local water as contaminated and as a preventive measure boiling tap water before drinking, brushing teeth and making ice cubes is highly recommended (Iamat, 2018).

Ethiopia is among the 5 countries that account for > 50% of all rotavirus deaths worldwide (DCP-3, 2013). The country has one of the highest prevalence of rotavirus globally, and is considered to have 6 percent of all deaths due to the viral infection (UNICEF, 2013).

Generally, about 88% of diarrhea-associated deaths are attributed to unsafe water, inadequate sanitation and insufficient hygiene (UNICEF, 2006; Black *et al.*, 2003).

Most reports showed the presence of rotavirus in Kenya among Kenyan population (Agutu *et al.*, 2017; Jacqueline *et al.*, 2009; Mohammad *et al.*, 2017). The routes of infection were reported to be fecal-oral transmission of the pathogen through contaminated drinking water (Saidi *et al.*, 1997).

Similarly, in Congo where rotavirus infection is common among children of age less than 60 months (Gontran *et al.*, 2016) with 23% prevalence among hospitalized children suffering from diarrhea (Cunliffe *et al.*, 1998).

Reports for Rwanda showed that diarrhea is the third cause of death among children especially for those who don't receive vaccination (Habtu *et al.*, 2017). This was attributed to insufficient supply of water and sizeable number of the people relying on contaminated water in the country (Dieudonné *et al.*, 2014).

In Uganda the virus was detected in 61% of the water samples collected from slum environment (Katukiza *et al.*, 2013). On the other hand, no reports were obtained for both Burundi and Tanzania

Vaccine Availability: Two brands of rotavirus Vaccines are now available, RotaTeq (RV5) and Rotarix (RV1). Babies receive either two or three doses depending on the type of vaccine administered. In case of RotaTeq, three doses are required at ages 2, 4, and 6 months whereas only two doses of Rotarix are required at ages of 2 and 4 months (CDC, 2018a) (WebMed, 2018).

In countries like Rwanda, Tanzania and Ethiopia, introducing rotavirus vaccine in 2013 lowered proportion of rotavirus positive hospitalizations between 2013–2015 as compared to other countries that had not introduced rotavirus vaccine. The decrease in rotavirus positivity was inversely related to increase in rotavirus vaccine coverage showing impact of rotavirus vaccination (Weldegebrei *et al.*, 2017).

Single Stranded RNA Viruses

(a) *Astrovirus*

Classification and Characteristics: Astrovirus belongs to the family Astroviridae. It is non-enveloped single stranded RNA virus (Matsui *et al.*, 2001).

Pathogenesis: Presence of viral particles both in fecal matter and in epithelial intestinal cells indicates that the virus replicates in the gastrointestinal tract of humans (Antimicrobe, 2016). The main symptoms are diarrhea, followed by nausea, vomiting, fever, malaise and abdominal pain (Bosch, 2014).

Gastroenteritis is usually caused by astrovirus infection. This results in destruction of the intestinal epithelial cells causing inhibition to absorption, loss of secretory functions, and decrease in permeability of the intestinal epithelia (Bosch, 2014).

Prevalence in River Nile Basin Countries: Not too many reports were found for detection of astrovirus in River Nile basin countries. In Egypt, the virus was found in 14% (Zaki and Abo El Kheir, 2017) and in another study in 17% of children (Abdollah *et al.*, 2000). In a report dealing with Egyptian children between 1 month and 18 years old, 1.7% of the fecal samples were positive for astrovirus (Kamel *et al.*, 2009). In Egypt, the virus was isolated from both the Nile and drinking water samples from areas in Giza and Maadi (El-Senousy *et al.*, 2007).

Astrovirus infection was detected both in Kenya (Caroline *et al.*, 2015; Shioda *et al.*, 2016; Nicholas *et al.*, 2007) and Tanzania (Samuel *et al.*, 2016; Saad *et al.*, 2018). But no reports were found from Sudan, Eritrea, Ethiopia, Congo, Burundi and Uganda.

Vaccine Availability: There is no available vaccine against Human astrovirus.

(b) *Norovirus*

Classification and Characteristics: Single-stranded RNA, non-enveloped viruses that belongs to the Caliciviridae family and sometimes referred to as the winter vomiting bug. The virus is not only spread by the fecal-oral route via contaminated food or water or person-to-person contact but also through the air (Brunette, 2017).

Pathogenesis: It is the most common cause of gastroenteritis (CDC, 2017). Infection is characterized by diarrhea, vomiting and stomach pain.

Symptoms usually develop 12 to 48 hours after infection, sometimes weakness, muscle aches, headaches and low-grade fevers may occur. Although, developing infection are unpleasant but norovirus is not usually dangerous. It is self-limiting and a person might reach complete recovery within two to three days from symptoms development (CDC, 2018b).

Prevalence in River Nile Basin Countries: Norovirus was detected in most of River Nile basin countries. In Egypt, a study reported that the virus was detected in 30% of Egyptian children (Zaki and Abo El Kheir, 2017) and in other reports the virus was detected in Egyptian children with different percentages (25.5%, 16.2%, and 9% respectively) (El-Nady *et al.*, 2014; Zaghloul *et al.*, 2013; El-Mohammady *et al.*, 2012) and detection was not limited to clinical samples but extended to drinking water (Sobsey *et al.*, 1988).

In Eritrea, it is recommended for all travelers that all local water should be considered contaminated. Recommendations were also made to boil tap water used for drinking, brushing teeth, and making ice cubes before use (Iamat, 2018), but no reports were found for Norovirus detection.

The virus was detected in infected hospitalized children in Ethiopia (Yassin *et al.*, 2012), Rwanda (Kabayiza *et al.*, 2013; Kabayiza *et al.*, 2014) and also Tanzania (Jean *et al.*, 2016).

In Kenya, the virus was detected in population (Shioda *et al.*, 2016, Nakata *et al.*, 1998) especially among children (Schilling *et al.*, 2010, Ahenda *et al.*, 2012) and also samples from the Nile water (Kiulia *et al.*, 2010).

For Sudan, Congo, Burundi no reports were found.

Vaccine Availability: There is no available vaccine for Norovirus.

(c) *Hepatitis A Virus*

Classification and Characteristics: It is not enveloped and contains a single-stranded RNA packaged in a protein shell. It belongs to family Picornaviridae (Cristina and Costa-Mattioli 2007). The virus spreads by the fecal–oral route infecting the liver (CDC, 2011). The virus is stable at pH 3 and resists a temperature of 60°C for 10 hours (Percival *et al.*, 2004). It remains stable after storage at room temperature and in water, sewage and shellfish for months (Sobsey *et al.*, 1988).

Pathogenesis: Symptoms usually last less than 2 months, although some people can be ill for as long as 6 months (CDC, 2011).They include fatigue, fever, nausea, loss of appetite, jaundice, a yellowing of the skin, bile moves from bloodstream and excreted in urine giving it a dark color, diarrhea, light, or clay-colored feces (acholic feces) and abdominal discomfort.

Prevalence in River Nile Basin Countries: The virus was detected in Egypt both in drinking (Ali *et al.*, 2004) and sewage water (Hamza *et al.*, 2017). Many outbreaks among European travelers returning from Egypt have been previously reported (Bernard and Frank, 2009; Couturier, 2009; Frank *et al.*, 2004). The largest of these was 350 cases of HAV infections that appeared among travelers from nine European countries returning from Egypt in 2004 and the reason for this was reported to be orange juice (Frank *et al.*, 2004). Infection was reported also among Egyptians (Salama *et al.*, 2007; Al-Aziz and Awad, 2008; Ali, 2002).

In Sudan, during the floods of 1988 in Khartoum, studies conducted on patients with acute hepatitis showed that 5.45% were infected with HAV (McCarthy *et al.*, 1994). Another study among children with acute hepatitis in Khartoum concluded that HAV was the cause of 33.3% of acute clinical hepatitis (Hyams *et al.*, 1992).

HAV antibody was detected in Ethiopia with prevalence rates 84 and 50% (Tsega *et al.*, 1992, Tsega 1986) respectively among the general population and children. The same was found in Kenya where HAV comes second after HBV with prevalence of 5 to 9% among different cities. Another report for Kenyan population showed that by the age of 14 about 77.6% received HAV infection (Sheila *et al.*, 2017).

In Burundi, a small study was made on 129 patients showed prevalence of 97.7% for HAV (Sheila *et al.*, 1997). In Uganda, the virus was recovered from 17% of water samples collected from poor environments (Katukiza *et al.*, 2013). In Tanzania the CDC recommended vaccination to all travelers with HAV vaccine (CDC, 2018c). Eritrea and Congo had no reports on HAV infection.

Vaccine Availability: Two types of HAV vaccines are currently internationally available, the live attenuated vaccine (based on H2 or LA-1 HAV strains) and the formaldehyde inactivated HAV vaccine which is used in most countries (WHO, 2018).

Vaccination is recommended for those who are at increased risks of exposure (such as from injecting drug use, oral-anal sex, travel to or residence in endemic areas, frequent clotting factor or blood transfusions) or with increased risks of fulminant disease (such as those with chronic hepatitis).

(d) *Hepatitis E Virus*

Classification and Characteristics: HEV is a positive-sense, single-stranded, non-enveloped, RNA icosahedral virus belonging to family Hepeviridae (Emerson *et al.*, 2012).

Pathogenesis: Infection with HEV has an incubation period varying between three to eight weeks before appearance of symptoms which may include jaundice, fatigue, and nausea. It correlates with elevated hepatic amino transferase levels (Emerson *et al.*, 2012).

Prevalence in River Nile Basin Countries: In Egypt, HEV is considered as a significant cause of acute viral hepatitis among Egyptian children (Gamal *et al.*, 2016) however, its incidence was reported very low in Nile water samples (1 of 72 samples; El-Senousy *et al.*, 2014) and the same was found on testing stool samples where HEV detection was not as predominant as HAV (Kamei *et al.*, 2011).

Conversely, in Sudan, during the floods of 1988 in Khartoum, studies on patients with acute hepatitis showed that infections were mainly HEV

(58%) with low incidence of HAV infection (5.45%; McCarthy *et al.*, 1994). Children suffering from acute hepatitis in Khartoum were found to be commonly infected with HEV (59% prevalence; Hyams *et al.*, 1992). Another large documented outbreak was reported from Mornay camp in western Darfur in 2004, where 2621 persons were found infected with HEV, with an attack rate of 3.3% out of a total population of 78,800 people, and an overall case-fatality rate of 1.7%. Death rate was high among pregnant women with a mortality rate of 31%. The virus was transmitted through drinking chlorinated surface water. It was thought that although levels of free residual chlorine in tap water were sufficient to reduce fecal coliform load, it may not have been enough to inactivate HEV (Guthmann *et al.*, 2006, Boccia *et al.*, 2006).

Infection was reported in Ethiopia among pregnant women (Tsega *et al.*, 1993; Abebe *et al.*, 2017), 93% in acute hepatitis patients and 3% of healthy controls (Tsega *et al.*, 1991a). HEV outbreaks were reported not only in Ethiopia (Tsega *et al.*, 1991b) but also in Kenya, Sudan, Uganda and Democratic Republic of Congo (Adelabu *et al.*, 2017).

In Burundi HEV infection was reported in a small study which included 123 patients and prevalence was found to be 14% (Aubry *et al.*, 1997). No more reports were found for the rest of the River Nile basin countries.

Vaccine Availability: Only one vaccine called Hecolin was licensed in China in December 2011 for use in people aged > 16 years. It is recommendded by the manufacturer for individuals at high risk of HEV infection, including those involved in animal husbandry, food handlers, students, members of the armed forces, women of childbearing age, as well as travelers to endemic areas (Innovax, 2014).

(e) *Enteroviruses*

Classification and Characteristics: They are non-enveloped single-stranded RNA viruses belonging to family Picornaviridae (King *et al.*, 2000). Enteroviruses are transmitted through the intestine thus the name 'enteroviruses'.

The enteroviruses include polioviruses, coxsackie A viruses (CA), coxsackie B viruses (CB), and echoviruses (Oberste *et al.*, 1999).

Pathogenesis

e.1. *Poliovirus:* The virus can survive in the acidic pH of the stomach, allowing its spread throughout the body via the lymphatic system (Goodsell, 1998).

Infection occurs via fecal-oral route and viral replication occurs in the tissues and muscles of the alimentary canal. Virus is shed in feces of infected persons and in 95% of the cases the virus is present in the blood stream. Infection is asymptomatic in 5% of cases. As the virus replicates and reaches the bloodstream, most of the symptoms appear including fever, headache and sore throat. Less than 1% of polio-infected cases suffer from paralytic poliomyelitis. The disease occurs when the virus enters the central nervous system and replicates in the motor neurons of the spinal cord, brain stem, or motor cortex leading to selective destruction of motor neurons and subsequently temporary or permanent paralysis.

Vaccine Availability: Two types of poliovirus vaccines are available the first is the inactivated polio vaccine which is the only polio vaccine that has been administered in the United States since 2000. It is given by shot in the arm or leg, depending on the person's age. The second vaccine is oral polio vaccine which is used in other countries.

CDC recommends that children receive four doses at each of the following ages:

- 2 months old
- 4 months old
- 6 through 18 months old
- 4 through 6 years old.

Almost all children (99 out of 100) who receive the recommended doses will be protected from polio (CDC, 2018d).

e.2. *Coxsackie A Viruses:* In general, group A coxsackie viruses tend to infect skin and mucous membranes, causing herpangina, acute hemorrhagic conjunctivitis and hand, foot, and mouth (HFM) diseases (Seitsonen *et al.*, 2012).

Vaccine Availability: There is no available vaccine for coxsackie A viruses.

e.3. *Coxsackie B viruses:* Group B coxsackie viruses tend to infect heart, pleura, pancreas, and liver causing pleurodynia, myocarditis, pericarditis and hepatitis (inflammation of the liver not related to the hepatotropic viruses). Coxsackie B infection of the heart can lead to pericardial effusion (Triantafyllopoulou *et al.*, 2004).

Vaccine Availability: There is no available vaccine forcoxsackie B viruses.

e.4. *Echovirus:* Echoviruses are common human pathogens that cause a range of illnesses ranging from minor febrile illness to severe, potentially fatal conditions (e.g. aseptic meningitis, encephalitis, paralysis and myocarditis) (Nino Khetsuriani *et al.*, 2005).

Vaccine availability: There is no available vaccine for Echovirus.

Prevalence of Enteroviruses in River Nile Basin Countries: In Egypt, a study recorded presence of enteroviruses in stool samples of school children and the highest prevalence was seen for Echovirus (Afifi *et al.*, 2009). Sequencing of detected enterovirus in drinking water samples was shown to be Cox B (El-Senousy *et al.*, 2017). An earlier study showed that 12% of the water samples contained enterovirus that was found to be poliovirus when sequenced (Shoeib *et al.*, 2009). Nile water samples collected showed 8 positive tests of which 87.5% contained poliovirus and 12.5% contained Cox B (Ali *et al.*, 1999).

In Sudan, a total of 53% of diabetic patients were Cox antibody positive (Emad *et al.*, 2011). In Sudan and Congo, although sharp decreases in acute flaccid paralysis resulting from poliovirus was observed, incidence increased again due to incomplete vaccine coverage, migration and limited public health systems (Infectious diseases advisor, 2018). Enteroviruses were detected in Congo and Burundi (Richter *et al.*, 2013, Piralla *et al.*, 2015) and Cox B virus in Kenya (Silvanos *et al.*, 2016). No reports were found about the epidemiology of enteroviruses in Eritrea, Ethiopia, Uganda and Tanzania.

Table 1: Viruses Circulating in the River Nile Basin Countries and Transmitted by Fecal-Oral Route

Country	*Circulating Viruses*
Egypt	Adenoviruses, Rotavirus, Astrovirus, Noroviruses, Hepatitis A Virus, Hepatitis E Virus, Enteroviruses
Sudan and South Sudan	Adenoviruses, Rotavirus, Hepatitis A Virus, Hepatitis E Virus, Enteroviruses
Eritrea	Rotavirus, Noroviruses
Ethiopia	Rotavirus, Noroviruses, Hepatitis A Virus, Hepatitis E Virus
Kenya	Adenoviruses, Rotavirus, Astrovirus, Noroviruses, Hepatitis A Virus, Hepatitis E Virus, Enteroviruses
Congo	Adenoviruses, Rotavirus, Hepatitis E Virus, Enteroviruses
Burundi	Hepatitis A Virus, Hepatitis E Virus, Enteroviruses
Rwanda	Rotavirus, Noroviruses
Uganda	Adenoviruses, Rotavirus, Hepatitis A Virus, Hepatitis E Virus
Tanzania	Adenoviruses, Astrovirus, Noroviruses, Hepatitis A Virus

Table 2: Available Vaccines for Water Transmitted Viruses

Virus	*Vaccine Availability*
Adenovirus	Adenovirus vaccine available, it contains live adenovirus Type 4 and Type 7
Rotavirus	Two brands of Rotavirus Vaccines are now available, RotaTeq (RV5) and Rotarix (RV1), two or three doses are administered according to vaccine type with RotaTeq, three doses are required. They should be given at ages 2 months, 4 months, and 6 months. Rotarix only requires two doses at 2 months and 4 months.
Astrovirus	No available vaccine
Norovirus	No available vaccine
Hepatitis A Virus	Two types of HAV vaccines that are currently available internationally, the live attenuated vaccine (based on H2 or LA-1 HAV strains and manufactured as well as mainly used in China and/or India) and the formaldehyde inactivated HAV vaccine which is used in most countries
Hepatitis E Virus	Only one vaccine called Hecolin was licensed in China in December 2011
Poliovirus	Two types of poliovirus vaccines are available the first is the Inactivated polio vaccine (IPV) which is the only polio vaccine that has been given in the United States since 2000. It is given by shot in the arm or leg, depending on the person's age. The second vaccine is Oral polio vaccine (OPV) which is used in other countries.
Coxsackie A Viruses	No available vaccine
Coxsackie B Viruses	No available vaccine
Echovirus	No available vaccine

4. CONCLUSIONS

The eleven (11) River Nile basin countries; Tanzania, Uganda, Rwanda, Burundi, the Democratic Republic of the Congo, Kenya, Ethiopia, Eritrea, South Sudan, Sudan and Egypt depend on the Nile for source of water. At the same time due to the low economic status of nearly all the said countries and the unavailability of water treatment plants, sewage water is dumped untreated and thus, represents the source of contaminants including viruses to the human populations.

Presence of nearly all the known water-borne viruses was reported in some of the River Nile basin countries namely; Egypt, Sudan and Kenya while limited information is available for Eritrea and Rwanda, this may be attributed to the absence of active surveillance programs to detect presence of viruses that might be circulating there.

Currently, vaccines are available to some of the water-borne viruses namely; adenovirus, rotavirus, poliovirus and HAV. Hepatitis E Virus (HEV) vaccine is only licensed for use in China. In case of astrovirus, norovirus, coxsackie A viruses, coxsackie B viruses and Echovirus no vaccines are available yet.

ACKNOWLEDGMENTS

The authors acknowledge the Egyptian Academy of Scientific Research and Technology for initiating the collaboration with the Centre for Science and Technology of the Non-Aligned and other Developing Countries and the National Research Center of Egypt for approving the collaboration and for providing all the logistics and facilities for preparing the chapter.

REFERENCES

[1] Abd El-Hady, H.H. (2014). Alternations in biochemical structures of phytoplankton in Aswan Reservoir and River Nile. Egypt. J. Biol. Environ. Sci. 4 (2):68–80.

[2] Abdollah, B., Naflcy, M.R., Rao. J.L., Holmes, T.F., Wierzba, R.W., Frenck, S.S., Monroe, R.I., Glass, J.D.C. (2000). Astrovirus Diarrhea in Egyptian Children .The Journal of Infectious Diseases, 182(3): 685–690.

[3] Abebe, M., Ali, I., Ayele, S., Overbo, J., Aseffa, A., Mihret, A. (2017): Seroprevalence and risk factors of Hepatitis E Virus infection among pregnant women in Addis Ababa, Ethiopia. PLoS One.12(6).

[4] Adelabu, O.A., ChuksIweriebor, B., Nwodo, U.U., Obi, L.C., Okoh, A.I. (2017). Incidence and molecular characterization of Hepatitis E virus from Swine in Eastern Cape, South Africa.AdvVirol. 1073253. doi: 10.1155/2017/1073253.

[5] Afifi, S.S. Zaki, S.A. Mohamed, A.F. and El Hosseiny, H. (2009). Isolation and identification of Non-Polio Enteroviruses from children in different Egyptian governorates. Australian Journal of Basic and Applied Sciences, 3(4): 3230–3238.

[6] Agutu, M.J., Ongus, J., Kombich, J., Kamenwa, R., Nyangao, J., Kagira, J., Ogutu, A.A., and Bitek, A. (2017). Prevalence and genetic diversity of rotavirus infection in children with acute gastroenteritis in a hospital setting, Nairobi Kenya in post vaccination era: a cross-sectional study, PanAfr Med J, 26: 38.

[7] Ahenda, P., Ng'ang'a, Z. and Panchalingam, S. (2012). Viral etiologies of diarrhea among children attending lwak mission hospital in Asembo, western Kenya. Am J Trop Med Hyg, 89 (l): 228–304.

[8] Ahmed, S.F., Mansour, A.M., Klena, J.D., Husain, T.S., Hassan, K.A., Mohamed, F. and Steele, D. (2014). Rotavirus genotypes associated with acute diarrhea in Egyptian infants. Pediatr Infect Dis J. 33 (1):62–68.

[9] Aimee, M. G., Benito, J. M., Yi, L., Joanna, L. S. (2015). Waterborne viruses: A Barrier to safe drinking water. PLoSPathog. 11(6).

[10] Al-Aziz, A.M. and Awad, M. A. (2008). Seroprevalence of hepatitis A virus antibodies among a sample of Egyptian children. EastMediterr Health J. 14(5): 1028–35.

[11] Ali, M.A. (2002). Partial sequence at 2BC region of HAV isolated from stool of acute sporadic HAV patients. J Egypt Public Health Assoc. 77(1–2):101–16.

[12] Ali, M.A., El-Esnawy, N.A., Shoaeb, A.R., Ibraheim, M., El-Hawaary, S.E. (1999). RT-PCR and cell culture infectivity assay to detect enteroviruses during drinking water treatment processes. J Egypt Public Health Assoc. 74(5–6): 651–61.

[13] Ali, M.A., Al-Herrawy, A.Z. and El-Hawaary, S.E. (2004). Detection of enteric viruses, Giardia and Cryptosporidium in two different types of drinking water treatment facilities. Water Res. 38(18):3931–9.

[14] Antimicrobe (2016). Astroviruses – Infectious Disease and Antimicrobial Agents. *www.antimicrobe.org*. Retrieved 2016-10–15.

[15] Aubry, P., Niel, L., Niyongabo, T., Kerguelen, S. and Larouze, B. (1997). Seroprevalence of hepatitis E virus in an adult urban population from Burundi. *Am J. Trop Med Hyg.* 57(3):272–3.

[16] Bernard, H. and Frank, C. (2009). Cluster of hepatitis A cases among travellers returning from Egypt, Germany, September through November 2008. Euro Surveill, 14(3).

[17] Bernstein, D.I. (2009). Rotavirus overview. The Pediatric Infectious Disease Journal. 28 (3): 50–53.

[18] Black, R.E., Morris, S., Bryce, J. (2003). Where and why are 10 million children dying every year? Lancet, 361(9376):2226–34.

[19] Boccia, D., Guthmann, J.P., Klovstad, H. (2006). High mortality associated with an outbreak of hepatitis E among displaced persons in Darfur, Sudan. Clin Infect Dis. 42:1679–84.

[20] Bosch, Albert (2014). Human Astroviruses. Clinical Microbiology Reviews. 27 (4): 1048.

[21] Britannica (2017): Lake Victoria. Encyclopaedia Britannica. https://www.britannica.com/place/Lake-Victoria 2017.

[22] Brunette, G. W. (2017). CDC Yellow Book 2018: Health information for international Travel. Oxford University Press. *p. 269.* ISBN 9780190628611.

[23] Butz, A.M., Fosarelli, P., Dick, J., Cusack, T., Yolken, R. (1993). Prevalence of rotavirus on high-risk fomites in day-care facilities. Pediatrics, 92 (2): 202–205.

[24] Caroline, T., Meyer, I.K., Bauer, M.A., Mitchell, A., Debasish, S., Joseph, O.O., John, B.O., Richard O., Colin, S. and Lori, R.H. (2015). Prevalence of classic, MLB-clade and VA-clade Astroviruses in Kenya and The Gambia Virol J. 12: 78.

[25] CDC (2011). "Hepatitis A Information for the Public". Center for Disease Control and prevention. *2009-09-17.* Archived from the original on 2011-05-22. Retrieved 2011-01-08.

[26] CDC (2014). Vaccine information statements. Center for Disease Control and prevention. https://www.cdc.gov/vaccines/hcp/vis/vis-statements/adenovirus.html. 6-11-2014.

[27] CDC (2018a). vaccine information statements. Center for Disease Control and prevention. https://www.cdc.gov/vaccines/hcp/vis/vis-statements/rotavirus.html. 23.2.2018.

[28] CDC (2018b). Norovirus. Center for Disease Control and prevention. https://www.cdc.gov/norovirus/hcp/clinical-overview.html. 1-6-2018.

[29] CDC (2018c). Health information for travellers to Tanzania. Center for Disease Control and prevention https://www.cdc.gov/travel/destinations/traveler/none/tanzania.2018.

[30] CDC (2018d). Vaccines and preventable diseases. Center for Disease Control and prevention. https://www.cdc.gov/vaccines/vpd/polio/index.html. 4-5-2018.

[31] Chen, Z.Q. Xiang, Y. Li, R.K. Kurupati, B. Jia, A. Bian, D.M. Zhou, N. Hutnick, S. Yuan, C. Gray, J. Serwanga, B. Auma, P. Kaleebu, X. Zhou, M. R. Betts and H.C.J. Ertl. (2010). Adenovirus-based vaccines: comparison of vectors from three species of *Adenoviridae*, J Virolv. 84(20).

[32] Couturier, E. (2009). Cluster of cases of hepatitis A with a travel history to Egypt, September - November 2008, France. Euro Surveill, 14(3).

[33] Cristina, J., Costa-Mattioli, M. (2007). "Genetic variability and molecular evolution of hepatitis A virus". Virus Res. 127 (2): 151–7.

[34] Cunliffe, N.A., Kilgore, P.E., Bresee, J.S., Steele, A.D., Luo, N. Hart, C.A. and Glass R.I. (1998). Epidemiology of rotavirus diarrhoea in Africa: a review to assess the need for rotavirus immunization. Bull World Health Organ. 76(5): 525–537.

[35] DCP-3 (2013). Diarrhea and rotavirus ECEAs for Ethiopia. Disease control priorities. Economic evaluation for health. http://www.dcp-3.org/sites/default/files/resources/ECEA_RV_diarrhea.pdf. 21-6-2013.

[36] Demian, P.N., Horton, K.C., Kajon, A., Siam, R., Hasanin, A.M.N., AmanyElgoharySheta, A.E., Cornelius, C. and Gaynor, A.M. (2014). Molecular identification of adenoviruses associated with respiratory infection in Egypt from 2003 to 2010. BMC Infect Dis. 14: 50.

[37] Dennehy, P.H. (2000). Transmission of rotavirus and other enteric pathogens in the home. *Pediatric Infectious Disease Journal,* 19 (10): 103–105.

[38] Dennehy, P.H. (2015). Rotavirus Infection: A disease of the past. Infectious Disease Clinics of North America, 29 (4): 617–35.

[39] Dieudonné, U., Cosmas, H.S. and Caroline, W.K. (2014). Prevalence and correlates for diarrhoea in the mountainous informal settlements of Huye town, Rwanda, Springerplus, 3: 745.

[40] Ecomena (2017). Egypt's water crisis, Recepie for disaster. EcoMEN. A https://www.ecomena.org/egypt-water/ 22-7-2017.

[41] El-Mohammady, H., Mansour, A., Shaheen, H.I., Henien, N.H., Motawea, M.S. and Raafat, I. (2012). Increase in the detection rate of viral and parasitic enteric pathogens among Egyptian children with acute diarrhea. J Infect Dev Ctries, 6(11):774–81.

[42] El-Nady, G.M., Badr, R.I., Salama, M.F., Shouman, B. and El-Bayoumi, M.A., 2014. Norovirus genogroup ii predominance in infants & young children with acute gastroenteritis in mansoura university children's hospital - Egypt. Pediatr Crit Care Med. 15(4):142.

[43] El-Sayed, M. and Salem, W.M. (2015). Hydrochemical assessments of surface Nile water and ground water in an industry area – South West Cairo. Egyptian Journal of Petroleum, 277–288.

[44] El-Senousy, W.M., Guix, S., Abid, I., Pintó, R.M. and Bosch A. (2007). Removal of Astrovirus from water and sewage treatment plants, evaluated by a competitive reverse transcription-PCR. Appl Environ Microbiol. 73(1): 164–167.

[45] El-Senousy, W.M., El-Gamal, M.S., Kamel, M.M. and El-Mahdy, E.M. (2014). Prevalence of human and animal Rotaviruses and HEV in Egyptian Nile water resources. World Applied Sciences Journal, 32 (11): 2218–2228.

[46] El-Senousy, W.M. Abdel-Moneim, A. Abdel-Latif, M. EL-Hefnawy, M. and Khalil, R.G. (2017). Coxsackievirus B4 as a causative agent of diabetes mellitus type 1: Is there a role of inefficiently treated drinking water and sewage in virus spreading? Food Environ Virol DOI 10.1007/s12560-017-9322-4

[47] Emad, M.A., Ali, Y.H., Enan, K.A. (2011). Epidemiology of Type 1 Diabetes mellitus among children in Sudan: Serological evidence of Coxsackievirus infection. *Journal of Science and Technology,* 12(4).

[48] Emerson, S.U., Purcell, R.H. Hepatitis, E. Virus. In: Knipe D.M., Howley, P.M., editors. *Fields Virology,* 5th. Vol. 392. Pennsylvania, Pa, USA: Lippincott Williams and Wilkins, 2007. pp. 3047–3058. *Hoofnagle, J. H.*, Nelson, K. E., Purcell, R. H. (2012): "Hepatitis E". New England Journal of Medicine. 367 (13): 1237–1244.

[49] Ezzat, S.M., Mahdy, H.M., Abo-State, M.A., Abd El Shakour, E.H. and El-Bahnasawy, M.A. (2012). Water quality assessment of River Nile at Rosetta Branch: impact of drains discharge. MEJSR 12 (4), 413– 423.

[50] FAO (2005). Eritrea. Food and agriculture organization of United Nations. http://www.fao.org/nr/water/aquastat/countries_regions/ERI/ 2005.

[51] Farthing, M.J.G. (1989). Gut viruses: A role in gastrointestinal disease. p. 1–4. In M. J. G. Farthing (ed.), Viruses and the gut. Smith Kline & French, Ltd., Welwyn Garden City, Hertfordshire, United Kingdom.

[52] Frank, C., Walter, J., Muehlen, M., Jansen, A., Treek, U., Hauri, A.M., Zoellner, I., Rakha, M., Hoehne, M., Hamouda, O., Schreier, E. and Stark, K. (2004). Major outbreak of hepatitis A associated with orange juice among tourists, Egypt, 2004.Emerg Infect Dis. 13(1): 156–158.

[53] Gamal, H., Asaad, A., Naglaa, M., Enas, D., Sayed, A., Ahmed, A., Ismail, M., Ayman, A., Ali, A. and Mohamad, H.T. (2016). Incidence and characteristics of hepatitis E virus infection in children in Assiut, *Upper Egypt J Int Med Res.* 44(5): 1115–1122.

[54] Goher, M.E., Hassan, A.M., Abdel-Moniem, I.A., Fahmy, A.H., ElSayed, S.M. (2014). Evaluation of surface water quality and heavy metal indices of Ismailia Canal, Nile River, *Egypt. Egypt. J. Aquat. Res.,* 40, 225–233.

[55] Gontran, M., Berge, N., Anissa, S., Victoire, M., Felix, K., Jeannhey, C.V., Sylvie, K.N., Thirumalaisamy, P.V. and Francine, N. (2016). Molecular epidemiology and surveillance of circulating rotavirus and adenovirus in Congolese children with gastroenteritis. *Journal of Medical Virology,* 88(4):596–605.

[56] Goodsell, D.S. (1998). The machinery of life. New York: Copernicus, ISBN 0-387-98273-6.

[57] Goshu, G., Koelmans, A.A., de Klein, J.J.M. (2017). Water quality of lake Tanabasin, Upper Blue Nile, Ethiopia. A review of available data. in: Stave K., Goshu G., Aynalem S. (eds) Social and Ecological System Dynamics. AESS Interdisciplinary Environmental Studies and Sciences Series. Springer, Cham.

[58] Guthmann, J.P., Klovstad, H. and Boccia, D. (2006). A large outbreak of hepatitis E among a displaced population in Darfur, Sudan, 2004: the role of water treatment methods. Clin Infect Dis. 42:1685–91.

[59] Habtu, M., Nsabimana, J. and Mureithi, C. (2017). Factors Contributing to Diarrheal Diseases among Children Less than Five Years in Nyarugenge District, Rwanda. *J. Trop Dis,* 5: 238.

[60] Hamza, H., Abd-Elshafy, D.N., Fayed, S.A., Bahgat, M.M., El-Esnawy, N.A., Abdel-mobdy, E. (2017). Detection and characterization of Hepatitis A virus circulating in Egypt. Arch. Virol. 162(7):1921–1931.

[61] Hashem, S., Shoman, S. A., Aly F. Mohamed, A.F. (2012). Isolation and molecular genotyping of group A Rotavirus strains circulating among Egyptian infants and children. Egyptian Journal of Medical Microbiology, 21(3):11–20.

[62] Hochwald, C. and Kivela, L. (1999). Rotavirus vaccine, live, oral, tetravalent (RotaShield). Pediatric Nursing. 25 (2): 203 207.

[63] Hogg, J. (2000). Latent adenoviral infection in the pathogenesis of emphysema. Chest, 117, 282–285.

[64] Hyams, K.C., Purdy, M.A. and Kaur, M. (1992). Acute sporadic hepatitis E in Sudanese children: analysis based on a new western blot assay. J Infect Dis., 165:1001–5.

[65] Iamat (2018). Eritrea. Food and water safety. https://www.iamat.org/country/eritrea/risk/food-water-safety-overview. 18-1-2018.

[66] Ibrahim, S.B., El-Bialy, A.A., Mohammed, M., El-Sheikh, A.O., Elhewala, A. and Bahgat, S. (2015). Detection of Rotavirus in children with acute gastroenteritis in Zagazig University Hospitals in Egypt. Electron Physician. 2015 Sep, 7(5): 1227–1233.

[67] Infectious disease advisor (2018): infectious disease: Enteroviruses including poliovirus, echovirus, coxsaxkievirus. infectious disease advisor. http://www.infectiousdiseaseadvisor.com/infectious-diseases/enteroviruses-including-poliovirus-echovirus-coxsackievirus/article/610264/ 2018.

[68] Innovax, 2014: Recombinant Hepatitis E Vaccine. Available at http://www.innovax.cn/en/pro1. aspx?CateID=52#103, accessed December 2014.

[69] Jacqueline, E., Tate Richard, D., Rheingans Ciara, E., O'Reilly, C. Burton, J.A., Tornheim (2009). Rotavirus disease burden and impact and cost-effectiveness of a Rotavirus vaccination program in Kenya, The Journal of Infectious Diseases, 200 (1): 76–84.

[70] Jean, P.K., Emma, M., Paul, R. H. and Natasha, P. (2016). Human Norovirus prevalence in Africa: a review of studies from 1990 to 2013 Tropical Medicine and International Health, 21(1): 2–17.

[71] Kabayiza, J.C., Andersson, M.E., Welinder-Olsson, C., Bergström, T., Muhirwa, G. and Lindh, M. (2013). Comparison of rectal swabs and faeces for real-time PCR detection of enteric agents in Rwandan children with gastroenteritis. BMC Infect Dis, 13, 447.

[72] Kabayiza, J.C., Andersson, M.E., Nilsson, S., Baribwira, C., Muhirwa, G., Bergström, T. and Lindh, M. (2014). Diarrhoeagenic microbes by real-time PCR in Rwandan children under 5 years of age with acute gastroenteritis. *Clin Microbiol Infect*, 20: 1128–1135.

[73] Kamel, A.H., Ali, M.A., El-Nady, H.G., de Rougemont, A., Pothier, P. and Belliot, G. (2009). Predominance and circulation of enteric viruses in the region of greater Cairo, *Egypt. J Clin Microbiol,* 2009, 47(4): 1037–1045.

[74] Kamel, A.H., Ali, M.A. El-Nagy, H.G., Deraz, A., Aho, S. and Pothier, P. (2011). Presence of enteric hepatitis viruses in the sewage and population of Greater Cairo. Clinical Microbiology and Infection. 17 (8), 1182–1185.

[75] Katukiza, A.Y., Temanu, H., Chung, J.W., Foppen, J.W., Lens, P.N. (2013). Genomic copy concentrations of selected waterborne viruses in a slum environment in Kampala, Uganda. *J. Water Health,* 11(2):358–70.

[76] King, A.M.Q., Brown, F., Christian, P., Hovi, T., Hyypiä, T., Knowles, N.J., Lemon, S.M., Minor, P.D., Palmenberg, A.C., Skern, T. and Stanway, G., 2000. Picornaviradae. In: Virus Taxonomy, Seventh Report of the International Committee for the Taxonomy of Viruses (ed. M.H.V. Van Regenmortel, C.M. Fauquet, D.H.L. Bishop, C.H. Calisher, E.B. Carsten, M.K. Estwes, S.M. Lemon, J. Maniloff, M.A. Mayo, D.J. McGeoch, C.R. Pringle and R.B. Wickner), pp. 657–673, Academic Press, New York, San Diego, USA.

[77] Kiulia, N.M., Netshikweta, R. and Page, N.A. (2010). The detection of enteric viruses in selected urban and rural river water and sewage in Kenya, with special reference to rotaviruses. *J Appl Microbiol,* 109: 818–828.

[78] Magzoub, A.M., Bilal, N.E., Bilal J.A. and Osman, O.F. (2013). Rotavirus infection among Sudanese children younger than 5 years of age: a cross sectional hospital-based study.PanAfr Med J. 16: 88.

[79] Matsui, S.M., Kiang, D., Ginzton, N., Chew, T., Geigenmüller-Gnirke, U., (2001). Molecular biology of astroviruses: Selected highlights. Novartis Found. Symp. Novartis Foundation Symposia. 238: 219–33, *"The Epidemiology of Astroviruses"*. web.stanford.edu. Retrieved 2016-10-15. https://www.youtube.com/watch?v=CtQYF3wlgL8.

[80] Mayindou, G., Ngokana, B., Sidibé, A., Moundélé, V., Koukouikila-Koussounda, F., Christevy Vouvoungui, J., Kwedi Nolna, S., Velavan, T.P. and Ntoumi, F. (2016). Molecular epidemiology and surveillance of circulating

rotavirus and adenovirus in Congolese children with gastroenteritis. Med Virol, 88(4):596–605.

[81] McCarthy, M.C., He, J., Hyams, K.C., el-Tigani, A., Khalid, I.O. and Carl, M. (1994). Acute hepatitis E infection during the 1988 floods in Khartoum, Sudan. Trans R Soc Trop Med Hyg. 88:177.

[82] Metzgar, D., Osuna, M., Yingst, S., Rakha, M., Earhart, K., Elyan, D., Esmat, H., Saad, M.D., Kajon, A., Wu, J., Gray, G.C., Ryan, M.A. and Russell, K.L. (2005). PCR analysis of Egyptian respiratory adenovirus isolates, including identification of species, serotypes, and coinfections. J Clin Microbiol. 43(11):5743–52.

[83] Mickan, L.D. and Kok, T.W. (1994). Recognition of adenovirus types in faecal samples by southern hybridization in South Australia. Epidemiology and Infection, 112(3), 603–613.

[84] Mohammad, S., Erick, O., Ernest, W., Cyrus, K., Martin, B., Gabriel, M., Sora, G., Satoshi, K., James, N. and Mohamed, K. (2017). Burden of Rotavirus and enteric bacterial pathogens among children under 5 Years of age hospitalized with diarrhea in suburban and rural Areas in Kenya Jpn. J. Infect. Dis., 70, 442–447.

[85] Moyo, S.J., Hanevik, K., Blomberg, B., Kommedal, O., Nordb, S.A., Maselle, S. and Langeland, N., 2014. Prevalence and molecular characterisation of human adenovirus in diarrhoeic children in Tanzania, a case control study BMC Infectious Diseases, 14:666.

[86] Naficy, A.B., Abu-Elyazeed, R., Holmes, J.L., Rao, M.R., Savarino, S.J., Kim, Y., Wierzba, T.F., Peruski, L., Lee, Y.J., Gentsch, J.R., Glass, R.I. and Clemens, J.D. (1999). Epidemiology of rotavirus diarrhea in Egyptian children and implications for disease control. Am J Epidemiol.150(7):770–7.

[87] Nakata, S., Honma, S. and Numata, K. (1998). Prevalence of human calicivirus infections in Kenya as determined by enzyme immunoassays for three genogroups of the virus. J ClinMicrobiol.36: 3160–3163.

[88] Nicholas, M., Kiulia, J.M., Mwenda, A.N., Julia, K., Nyaundi (2007). Astrovirus infection in young Kenyan children with Diarrhoea. Journal of Tropical Pediatrics, 53(3):206–209.

[89] Nilerak (2005). Http://nilerak.hatfieldgroup.com/English/NRAK/Resources/Document_centre/WQ_Baseline_report_Kenya.pdf .

[90] Nino Khetsuriani, M.D., Ashley LaMonte-Fowlkes, M.P.H., Steven O., Mark A.P. Enterovirus surveillance—United States, 1970–2005 MMWR surveillance summaries, September 15, 2006/55(SS08), 1–20

[91] Oberste, M.S., Maher, K., Kilpatrick, D.R., Pallansch, M.A. (1999). Molecular evolution of the human Enteroviruses: correlation of Serotype with VP1 sequence and application to Picornavirus classification. *J. Virol. 73 (3): 1941–8.*

[92] Oloo, A. (2007). The quest for cooperation in the Nile water conflicts: A Case for Eritrea, African Sociological Review. 11 (1).

[93] Onyango D.M. and Angienda P.O. (2010). Epidemiology of waterborne diarrhoeal diseases among children aged 6–36 months old in Busia – Western

Kenya. World Academy of Science, *Engineering and Technology International Journal of Environmental and Ecological Engineering,* 4 (1).

[94] Pauly, M., Hoppe, E., Mugisha, L., Petrzelkova, K., Akoua-Koffi, C., Couacy-Hymann E, Anoh, A.E., Mossoun, A., Schubert, G., Wiersma, L., Pascale, S., Muyembe, J.J., Karhemere, S., Weiss, S., Leendertz, S.A., Calvignac-Spencer, S., Leendertz, F.H. and Ehlers, B. (2014). High prevalence and diversity of species D adenoviruses (HAdV-D) in human populations of four Sub-Saharan countries. Virol J. 11, 11:25.

[95] Percival, S.L., Chalmer, R.M., Embrey, M., Hunter, P.R., Sellwood, J. and Wyn-Jones, P. (2004). Microbiology of waterborne diseases. Elsevier Academic Press, Great Britain. 480pp.

[96] Piralla, A., Daleno, C., Girello, A., Esposito, S. and Baldanti, F. (2015). Circulation of two Enterovirus C105 (EV-C105) lineages in Europe and Africa. *J Gen Virol.,* 96(6):1374–9.

[97] Rao, V.C., Melnick, J.L., 1986. Environmental virology. In: Cole, J.A., Knowles, C.J., Schlessinger, D. (eds) Aspects of Microbiology 13. Washington, D.C: American Society for Microbiology.

[98] Richter, J., Tryfonos, C., Panagiotoi, C., Nikolaou, E., Koliou, M., Christodoulou, C. (2013). Newly emerging C group enteroviruses may elude diagnosis due to a divergent 5′-UTR. International Journal of Infectious Diseases, 17(12): 1245–1248.

[99] Robesyn, E., Micalessi, M.I., Quoilin, S., Naranjo, M. and Thomas, I. (2009). Cluster of hepatitis A cases among travellers returning from Egypt, Belgium, September through November 2008. Euro Surveill, 14(3).

[100] Rosenbaun, H.C., chemical pollution and nutrient pollution/contaminants-urban, WWW.environment.gov.au/archive, retrieved 2/7/2013, 1994.

[101] Saad, B. Omer, Kristen Allen, D.H. Chang, L. Beryl Guterman, Robert A. Bednarczyk, Alex Jordan, Alison Buttenheim, Malia Jones, Claire Hannan, M. Patricia deHart, Daniel A. Salmon (2018). Exemptions from Mandatory Immunization after Legally Mandated Parental Counseling. Pediatrics, 141(1).

[102] Saidi, S.M., Iijima, Y., Sang, W.K., Mwangudza, A.K., Oundo, J.O., Taga, K., Aihara, M., Nagayama, K., Yamamoto, H., Waiyaki, P.G. and Honda, T., (1997). Epidemiological study on infectious diarrheal diseases in children in a coastal rural area of Kenya.MicrobiolImmunol, 41(10): 773–8.

[103] Salama, I.I., Samy, S.M., Shaaban, F.A., Hassanin, A.I., Abou Ismail, L.A. (2007). Seroprevalence of hepatitis A among children of different socio-economic status in Cairo. *East Mediterr Health J.,* 13(6):1256–64.

[104] Samuel, C., Francisco, B., Diem-Lan, V., Lara, T., Mary, K., Esther, K., Blaise, G., Evgeny, M.Z., Valérie, D., and Laurent, K., 2016. Astrovirus VA1 identified by next-generation sequencing in a nasopharyngeal specimen of a febrile Tanzanian child with acute respiratory disease of unknown etiology, Emerging Microbes &Infections, 5: e67

[105] Schilling, K.A., Omore, R. and Ayers, T., 2010. Characteristics and etiology of moderate-to-severe diarrhea of prolonged or persistent duration among

children less than five years old in rural western Kenya, 2008–2009. Am J Trop Med Hyg, 83 (5): 211–S282.

[106] Seitsonen, J., Shakeel, S., Susi, P., Pandurangan, A. P., Sinkovits, R.S., Hyvönen, H., Laurinmäki, P., Ylä-Pelto, J., Topf, M., Hyypiä, T. and Butcher, S.J. (2012). Structural analysis of coxsackievirus A7 reveals conformational changes associated with uncoating. Journal of Virology. 86 (13): 7207–7215.

[107] Shamrukh, M. and Abdel-Wahab, A. (2011). Water pollution and riverbank filtration for water supply along River Nile, Egypt. In: Shamrukh, M. (Ed.), Riverbank Filtration for Water Security in Desert Countries, Springer Science+Business Media B.V., 5–28.

[108] Sheila, M., Frédéric, L., Nadine, N., Steve, A., Richard, O., Berthold, B. M., Elisabeth, P., Athenaïs, G., Jessica, L.A., Dieudonné, M., Nicolas, B., Eric, M.L., Jean-Jacques, M. High prevalence and diversity of Hepatitis viruses in suspected cases of Yellow Fever in the Democratic Republic of Congo, J Clin Microbiol. 55(5): 1299–1312.

[109] Shioda, K., Cosmas, L., Audi, A., Gregoricus, N., Vinjé, J., Parashar, U.D., Montgomery, J.M., Feikin, D.R., Breiman, R.F. and Hall, A.J. (2016). Population-based incidence rates of diarrheal disease associated with Norovirus, Sapovirus, and Astrovirus in Kenya. PLoS One. 11(4).

[110] Shoeib, A.R., Abd El Maksoud, S.N., Barakat, A.B., Shoman S.A. and El-Esnawy, N.A. (2009). Comparative assessment of mammalian Reoviruses versus Enteroviruses as indicator for viral water pollution. J Egypt Public Health Assoc. 84(1–2):181–96.

[111] Silvanos, M. Opanda, Fred Wamunyokoli, Samoel, Khamadi, Rodney Coldren and Wallace, D. Bulimo Springerplus (2016). Genotyping of enteroviruses isolated in Kenya from pediatric patients using partial VP1 region. Springerplus, 5: 158.

[112] Sobsey, M.D., Shields, P.A., Hauchman, F.S., Davis, A.L., Rullman, V.A. and Bosch, A. (1988). Survival and persistence of hepatitis A virus in environmental samples. In: A. J. Zuckerman (ed) Viral hepatitis and liver diseases, pp. 121–124. New York: Alan R. Liss.

[113] Sudan W.I.E., Humodi A.S., Omer, E.E and Ali, A.S. (2013). Prevalence of rotavirus and adenovirus associated with diarrhea among displaced communities in Khartoum, BMC Infectious Diseases. 13:209.

[114] Tate, J.E., Burton, A.H. and Boschi-Pinto, C. (2008). Estimate of worldwide rotavirus associated mortality in children younger than 5 years before the introduction of universal rotavirus vaccination programmes: a systematic review and meta analysis. The Lancet Infectious Diseases, 12(2):136–141.

[115] Tate, J.E., Burton, A.H., Boschi-Pinto, C. and Parashar, U.D. (2016). Global, regional, and national estimates of rotavirus mortality in children < 5 years of age, 2000–2013. Clinical Infectious Diseases. 62(2): 96–105.

[116] Thacker, E.E., Nakayama, M., Smith, B.F., Bird, R.C., Muminova, Z., Strong, T.V., Timares, L., Korokhov, N., O'Neill, A.M., De Gruijl, T.D., Glasgow, J.N., Tani, K. and Curiel, D.T. (2009). A genetically engineered adenovirus vector targeted to CD40 mediates transduction of canine dendritic

cells and promotes antigen-specific immune responses in vivo. Vaccine. 27 (50): 7116–7124.

[117] Thompson, S.S., Jackson, J.L., Suva-Castillo, M., Yanko, W.A., El Jack, Z., Kuo, J.C.C., Williams, F.P. and Schnurr, D.P. (2003). Detection of infectious human adenoviruses in tertiary-treated and ultraviolet-disinfected wastewater. Water Environment Research: a Research Publication of the Water Environment Federation, 75(2), 163–170.

[118] Thurston-Enriquez, J.A., Haas, C.N., Jacangelo, J., Riley, K. and Gerba, C.P. (2003). Inactivation of feline calicivirus and adenovirus type 40 by UV radiation. Applied and Environmental Microbiology. 69(1), 577–582.

[119] Triantafyllopoulou, A., Tapinos, N. and Moutsopoulos, H. (2004). Evidence for Coxsackievirus infection in primary Sjogren's syndrome. American College of Rheumatology, 50(9): 2897–2902.

[120] Tsega, E., Mengesha, B. and Hansson, B.G. (1986). Hepatitis A, B, and delta infection in Ethiopia: a serologic survey with demographic data. Am J Epidemiol. 123(2): 344–51.

[121] Tsega, E., Krawczynski, K., Hansson, B.G., Nordenfelt, E., Negusse, Y., Alemu, W., Bahru, Y. (1991). Outbreak of acute hepatitis E virus infection among military personnel in northern Ethiopia. J Med Virol. 34(4):232–6.

[122] Tsega, E., Nordenfelt, E. and Hansson, B.G. (1992). Chronic liver disease in Ethiopia: a clinical study with emphasis on identifying common causes. Ethiop Med J. 30(2 Suppl):1–33.

[123] Tsega, E., Krawczynski, K., Hansson, B.G. (1993). Hepatitis E virus infection in pregnancy in Ethiopia. Ethiop Med J. 31(3):173–81.

[124] UNICEF (2013). Ethiopia launches rotavirus vaccine. UNICEF Ethiopia. https://www.unicef.org/esaro/5440_ethiopia_rotavirus-vaccine.html.8-11-2013.

[125] USAID (2006). Sudan water and sanitation profile. http://pdf.usaid.gov/pdf_docs/PNADO924.pdf

[126] Villena, C., El-Senousy, W.M., Abad, F.X., Pintó, R.M. and Bosch, A. (2003). Group A Rotavirus in sewage samples from Barcelona and Cairo: Emergence of unusual Genotypes. Appl Environ Microbiol. 69(7): 3919–3923.

[127] Wan and DeGregori (2000). Transgenic expression of the coxsackie/adenovirus receptor enables adenoviral-mediated gene delivery in naive T cells. Proc Natl Acad Sci USA. 2000 Dec 5, 97(25): 13784-9

[128] Webmd (2018). Rotavirus vaccine. WebMD. https://www.webmd.com/children/vaccines/rotavirus-rv-vaccine#1 2018.

[129] Weldegebrei, G., Mwenda, J.M., Chakauya, J., Daniel, F., Masresha, B., Parashar, U.D., E. Tale, J. (2017). Impact of rotavirus vaccine on rotavirus diarrhoea in countries of East and Southern Africa. Vaccine. 17:31458–5

[130] WHO (2011). Guidelines for drinking-water quality, 4th ed. Geneva, Switzerland: WHO Press.

[131] WHO (2014a). http://www.who.int/nuvi/surveillance/RV_bulletin_Jan_June_2012_Final.pdf. Accessed April 17, 2014 a.

[132] WHO (2014b). http://www.who.int/immunization/monitoring_surveillance/burden/estimates/rota virus/en/index.html. Accessed April 17, 2014 b.

[133] WHO (2018). International travel and health. Hepatitis A. World Health Organization. http://www.who.int/ith/vaccines/hepatitisA/en/ 2018.

[134] Yassin, M.A., Kirby, A. and Mengistu, A.A. (2012). Unusual norovirus and rotavirus genotypes in Ethiopia. Paediatr Int Child Health, 32: 51–55.

[135] Zaghloul, M.Z., El-Sahn, S.F. and Galal, Z.A. (2013). Coinfection of rotavirus group a, norovirus and adenovirus in Egyptian children with gastroenteritis. Life Sci J. 10(2):848–52.

[136] Zaki, M.E. and Abo El Kheir, N. (2017). Molecular study of astrovirus, adenovirus and norovirus in community acquired diarrhea in children: One Egyptian center study Asian Pac J Trop Biomed, 7(11): 987–990.

Subunit and Epitope-Based Vaccines against Shigelosis: Use of R-Lactobacilli for Antigen Delivery

Harish Padh[1] and Priti Desai[2]

[1]Sardar Patel University, Vallabh Vidhyanagar, Anand, Gujarat, India

[2]School of Biological Sciences & Biotechnology,
Institute of Advanced Research, Koba, Gandhinagar, Gujarat, India

E.mail: [1]hpadh@yahoo.com

ABSTRACT: Shigellosis, an infectious disease, spreads via contaminated food and water. It afflicts millions of people worldwide with an estimated one million fatalities per annum. Effective vaccine is one of the most promising approaches to fight against multidrug resistant Shigella. Despite extensive research during the last two decades, vaccine against Shigella is not available in the market. To provide cross protection against multiple Shigella strains, we selected outer membrane proteins OmpA and OmpC as candidate antigens. Both antigens were found to be conserved among Shigella as well as other enteric bacteria. Immunization with r-OmpA and r-OmpC successfully induced the systemic and cellular responses and protected the immunized Balb/C mice when challenged with S. flexneri. Furthermore, epitopes from both antigens were derived using advanced immunoinformatic tools. In vitro and in vivo validation of the selected epitopes indicated their critical role in activating host immune system. We have engineered r-L. lactis to deliver the DNA/protein at the mucosal sites and induce both mucosal and systemic immune responses. r-L. lactis expressing the OmpA gene were able to provide both systemic and mucosal immunity when orally administer to Balb/C mice. Immunized mice developed protection as revealed by surviving challenge infection with lethal Shigella strains, the survive ratios of mice immunized with rOmpA was 50% after 48 h post-challenge. Additionally, cytokine profiling (Th1 and Th2) revealed induction of cellular immunity upon vaccination. In general, the Th1 response is characterized by an increase in antigen-specific interferon-gamma (IFN-γ), IL-12, and complement-fixing antibodies, whereas the Th2 phenotype is characterized by production of IL-4, IL-5, IL-10, and an increase in IgE, IgA, and overall IgG antibodies. Simultaneously, newly constructed Shigella DNA vaccine was also delivered using r-L. lactis which successfully provoked significant increase in IgE, IgA, and overall IgG antibodies in response.

Keywords: Outer Membrane Proteins (OMP), Epitopes, DNA Vaccine, Lactococcus Lactis, Shigella, Mucosal Immunity, Protection, Humoral Immunity, Cellular Immunity.

1. INTRODUCTION

Shigellosis which is also known as bacterial dysentery is caused by the ingestion of *Shigella* spp. *via.* contaminated food and water. Once ingested, it initiates infection at colonic mucosal sites and leads to chronic inflammation and tissue damage followed by watery diarrhea along with severe abdominal pain and cramping. In severe cases, it results in bloody mucoid stool and cause fatality (Taneja 2007). It is estimated that *Shigella* causes 1.1 million deaths and 164. 7 million cases per annum worldwide (Mani *et al.,* 2016). Recent Global Enteric Multicenter Study (GEMS) which was performed in sub-Saharan Africa and South Asia confirmed that *Shigella* is a major cause of Moderate to Severe Diarrhea (MSD) in younger children (less than five years of age) and one of the top four causes of potentially life threatening diarrheal illness in both regions (Kotloff 2013). This study also indicates that MSD remains associated with significantly increased risk of mortality, cognitive defects and stunting. Oral rehydration therapy is not much more effective for shigellosis as it invades and destroys the mucosal lining further emergence of multidrug resistance *Shigella* spp. which worsens the conditions. Though this infection can be preventable by imposing standard hygiene conditions and safe drinking water, but providing both in the poor and crowded places is still unachievable. To prevent the *Shigella* infection and to fight against the anti-microbial resistance, vaccine is one of the cost effective alternatives. However, despite research for several decades, there is no single protective vaccine against *Shigella* available in the market (Mani *et al.,* 2016).

To design a new efficient vaccine against shigellosis, observations from natural infections and reasons for failure of various previous vaccine strategies are very important. *Shigella* invades and initiates its infection at mucosal sites, therefore, induction of both mucosal immunity and cellular immunity is very essential to develop protection (Sansonetti 2001). *Shigella spp.* is broadly divided into four major groups (*Shigella flexneri, Shigella boydii, Shigella sonnei* and *Shigella dysenteriae*) and 50 different serotypes (WHO 2006). The prevalence of them varies with both seasonally and geographically, study of infection pattern in Henan

Province, China, indicates that infections increased from May and reached highest number of infections in July (Xia *et al.,* 2011, Zhang *et al.,* 2011). Among them, *S. flexneri* is highly prevalent allover the world and responsible for most of the infections while *S. sonnei* is more common in low and middle income countries (Zaidi and Estrada-García 2014). *S. dysenteriae* is historically associated with epidemics in developing countries and refugee camps and *S. boydii* accounts only for less than 6% of total cases (Kotloff 2017). Therefore, a single vaccine, which can protect an individual from multiple strains of *Shigella* spp. and provide sufficient cellular, humoral and mucosal immunity is urgently needed.

With this background, our group is working to develop cost effective oral mucosal vaccine to provide protection against multiple serotypes of *Shigella*. In this chapter, we are summarizing our work which includes establishment of a new human like murine shigellosis model, identification and validation of conserved immunogenic antigens as well as their epitopes, engineering new food grade bacteria as an antigen (protein/ DNA) delivery vehicle by mucosal routes and evaluating the immunogenic and protective efficacies of the engineered bacterial strains.

2. HUMAN LIKE MURINE SHIGELLOSIS MODEL

One of the main reasons for the failure faced previous trials to elect effective vaccine candidates against *Shigella* so far is the lack of the appropriate animal models to study the disease pathology and to evaluate the vaccine efficacy (Levin *et al.,* 2007). Various animal models such as macaque monkey, rabbit, guinea pig and mice were previously used to understand pathogenesis of human shigellosis. Among them, mice model is getting an edge over others because its low cost, availability and ease of handling. However, adult mice don't develop human like shigellosis symptoms as they lack IL-8. Recruitment of neutrophils through secretion of IL-8 is one of the essential requirements for disease establishment (Phalipon and Sansonetti 2007). To establish a murine model for shigellosis '***SCID mouse-human intestinal xenograft model***' and "4-day old neonatal mice model" were developed (Zhang *et al.,* 2001). Both models have enormous potential, but their usage still remains not common due to laborious and lake of skilled expertise to maintain. In contrast, pulmonary infection of *Shigella* in intranasally (*i.n.*) challenged mice developed acute broncho pneumonia resulted in massive neutrophils infiltration which represents and simulates one of the major characteristics of shigellosis (Mallett *et al.,* 1993). Thus, this model is one of the widely used models in accessing vaccine efficacy, although it lacks the clinical relevance in the context of the site of infection (Phalipon and Sansonetti 2007). Recently, Yang and colleagues have established the shigellosis murine model by intraperitoneal (*i.p.*) infection, which mimics human shigellosis and seems promising in accessing potential vaccine candidates in the future (Yang *et al.,* 2014). In this line, we have also established a murine shigellosis model using intraperitoneal route and compared it with the previously accepted intranasal model (Sharma *et al.,* 2016). Simultaneously, we have also undertaken a comparative analysis of *i.n.* vs *i.p.* routes of administration with relatively high and low dose of infection to understand the appropriate dose and suitable route of administration to establish the appropriate model for evaluating immunogenicity and protective efficacy of prophylactic candidates.

We have used 6–8 weeks old Balb/C mice to compare the route of administration in the establishment of the shigellosis murine model. One group of mice received the *S. flexeneri* (ATCC 12022) *i.n.* and other group received it *i.p.* These groups were further divided into high dose (receiving 10^8 CFU of *S. flexneri*), low dose (receiving 10^6 CFU of *S. flexneri*) and saline control group (receiving PBS). Mice were kept for observations for 3 days before infection and 7 days after infection. Parameters such as general physical activity, change in physiological conditions (body temperature, body weight, rectal temperature, fur ruffling, abdominal swelling and conjunctivitis), consistency of stool and presence of mucus or blood in the feces were recorded. *Shigella* Shedding in the feces along with the colonization in the infected tissues (lung and colon) were also counted using the SS agar plating method. After 7 days of infection, both small and large intestine from *i.p.* challenged group and lung tissue from *i.n.* challenged animals were collected and subjected to haematoxylin and eosin (H&E) staining.

As seen from the Figure 1 and 2, dysentery like symptoms were observed in the *i.p.* group while, in the *i.n.* group only mild inflammatory symptoms restricted to the site of infection were observed. This might be due to the clinical irrelevance of the site of the infection. Among the i.p. group, mice who received the high dose exhibited severe dysentery, leading to 100% mortality within 18 hours of infection. On the contrary, low dose infection with *S. flexneri* (~10^6 CFU) induced diarrhea with mild inflammatory responses. Hence these results reflect the impact of both the site of infection and the infection dose on the disease outcomes to be considered while establishing a successful murine shigellosis model (Sharma *et al.,* 2016).

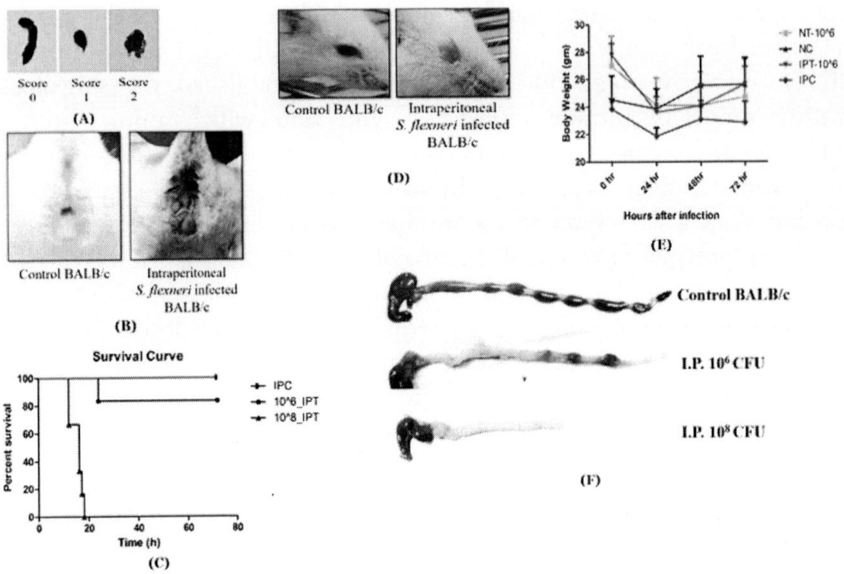

Fig. 1: *Shigella* pathogenesis in adult BALB/c mice after *i.p.* and *i.n.* infection, (A) Fecal morphological scoring based on stool consistency. (B) Photos of anal region of control and *i.p. S. flexneri* infected mice. (C) Graphical representation of survival rates of *i.p.* infected and control mice ($P < 0.0001$). (D) Photos of bacterial conjunctivitis induced in IPHD group of mice. (E) Graph representing change in body weight at different time points post infection. (F) Colon length of *i.p.* infected mice receiving low and high dose of *S. flexneri*.

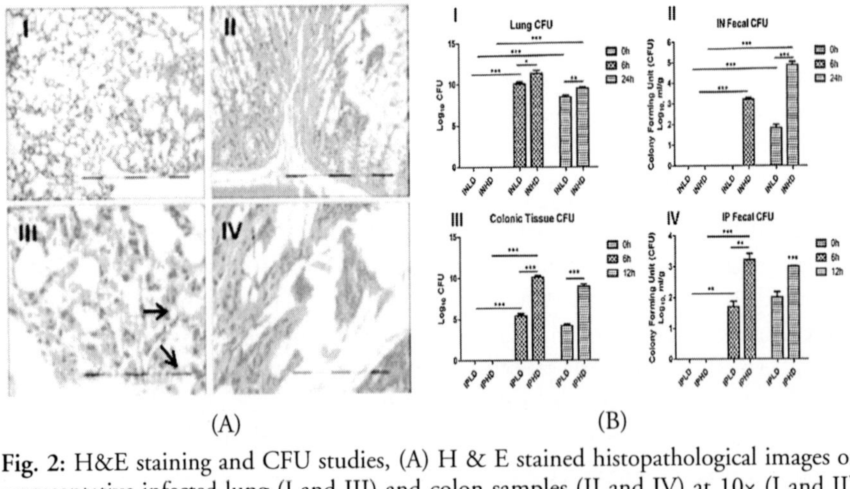

Fig. 2: H&E staining and CFU studies, (A) H & E stained histopathological images of representative infected lung (I and III) and colon samples (II and IV) at 10× (I and II) and 40× (III and IV) magnification. Arrow indicates the infiltrated PMN. (B) Colony-forming units (CFU) in homogenates of colon, lung and feces at 0, 6, 12 and 24 h post *i.p.* and *i.n.* infection with *Shigella*.

3. IDENTIFICATION AND VALIDATION OF ANTIGENS AND THEIR EPITOPES

Despite the significant burden of shigellosis, there is no single licensed vaccine available in the public domain. Shigellosis is caused by 4 different *Shigella* strains and more than 50 different serotypes. However, the protective response against *Shigella* is serotype specific (Sansonetti *et al.*, 2007) and hence the development of a multivalent vaccine capable of providing cross-protection against multiple strains is desirable. There are two basic approaches to attain protection against a wide range of *Shigella* spp; either by combining efficacious serotype-targeted antigens in a multivalent vaccine or by using a cross reactive antigen in the vaccine design. To identify the conserved antigens, OMPs (Outer Membrane Proteins) of all four *Shigella* spp. were isolated and characterized. The antisera raised against the OMPs of *S. flexneri* exhibited binding with the OMPs derived from other *Shigella* spp. in the Western blot analysis, which supports the conservancy of OMPs in all four *Shigella* spp. Further 2D PAGE analysis of OMPs reveled overexpression of the two outer membrane proteins i.e. OmpA and OmpC. A multiple sequence alignment analysis confirmed the conservancy of OmpA and OmpC in *Shigella* (~90%) and *Salmonella* (~75%). Also, we have identified epitopes from OmpA and OmpC of *Shigella* which are potent immunogens and found them conserved among all the *Shigella* spp. (Sharma 2018).

We have identified a pool of epitopes derived from OMPs of *Shigella* by rational deployment of immunoinformatic tools. With the aim to have common epitopes to generate humoral and cell mediated immunity, we derived T cell epitopes from B cell epitopes. The epitopes were screened through several selection criteria such as topological surface exposure, binding to maximum *Major Histocompatibility Complex (MHC)* alleles and high population coverage (Turbyfill *et al.*, 1995). Out of the predicted epitopes, high scoring epitopes derived from OmpA and OmpC were selected and experimentally validated (Sharma *et al.*, 2016). OmpA, OmpC and their potent epitopes were selected as candidate antigens and evaluated for their immunogenicity and protective efficacy using the above described inhouse developed murine shigellosis model.

4. EVALUATION OF THE IMMUNOGENICITY AND PROTECTIVE EFFICACY OF THE R-OMPA, R-OMPC AND THEIR POTENT EPITOPES

Gene sequences of the OmpA and OmpC proteins of *Shigella dysenteriae* type-1 (Accession number/Gene ID 3799631 and 946716 respectively) were retrieved from NCBI. Both genes were cloned into the pET28a vector. Proteins were expressed and purified from *E. coli* BL 21. Purified OmpA and OmpC recombinant proteins were then used to immunized Balb/C mice *via* intramuscular route. Both the proteins successfully induced significant serum IgG levels and cytokine responses like IL-6, IL-8, IL-4, IL-10 and gamma interferon (Data under communication).

5. DELIVERY OF ANTIGENS (PROTEINS/DNA) USING THE LIVE FOOD GRADE BACTERIA LACTOCOCCUS LACTIS (L. LACTIS)

Shigella, being an intracellular pathogen, initiates its infection by invading the colonic mucosa and establish the disease. Thus, both mucosal and systemic immune responses are desired to provide protection against infection. Previous attempts to developed oral mucosal vaccine used either attenuated strains or purified macromolecules. Attenuated approach, although generates mucosal immunity, it is limited to the strains used for its preparation and many times poses risks for reversion of pathogenicity. On the other hand, purified macromolecule in the form of a subunit vaccine is safe, but generates short live immune response and fails to provide mucosal immunity (Levin *et al.*, 2007). With this background, we developed a new vaccine delivery platform using *L. lactis,* a food grade bacteria. *L. lactis* is non-commensal, non-invasive, Gram positive bacteria which has been widely explored for oral delivery of antigens, antibodies and a variety of therapeutic proteins. Delivery through r-*L. lactis* has been shown to protect antigenic cargo from denaturing gastric environment and favor direct uptake into Peyer's patches which results in elicitation of systemic as well as mucosal immune response essential for successful elimination of enteric pathogens such as *Shigella* (Yagnik *et al.*, 2017).

5.1 L. Lactis as a Delivery Vehicle for Protein Antigen, OmpA

We have previously identified an outer membrane protein A (OmpA) of *Shigella dysenteriae* type-1 (SD-1) as a conserved antigen. The *ompA* gene was cloned by replacing nuclease gene in pSEC:Nuc vector under nisin inducible promoter and named pSEC:OmpA. Two different strains of *L. lactis* were transformed with pSEC:OmpA and studied for OmpA expression. Expression of OmpA in *L. lactis* was optimized using several factors such as host proteases, inducer concentration and precipitating agents. The developed r-*L. lactis* expressing OmpA (*LacVax®:OmpA*) strains were used to evaluate two different mucosal routes for their Immunogenicity. Oral route was found to be more promising compared to nasal route as oral administration of *LacVax®:OmpA* resulted in higher serum IgG and fecal IgA levels compared to nasal route of immunization (Figure 3) (Yagnik *et al.,* 2017). Further, Balb/C mice immunized orally with *LacVax®:OmpA* were challenged with *S. flexneri* in order to assess its protective efficacy. Pathophysiological characteristics such as absence of tissue destruction, low inflammation and moderate physical activities of vaccinated animals following *Shigella* challenge highlights the protective strength of the vaccine candidate (data in communication).

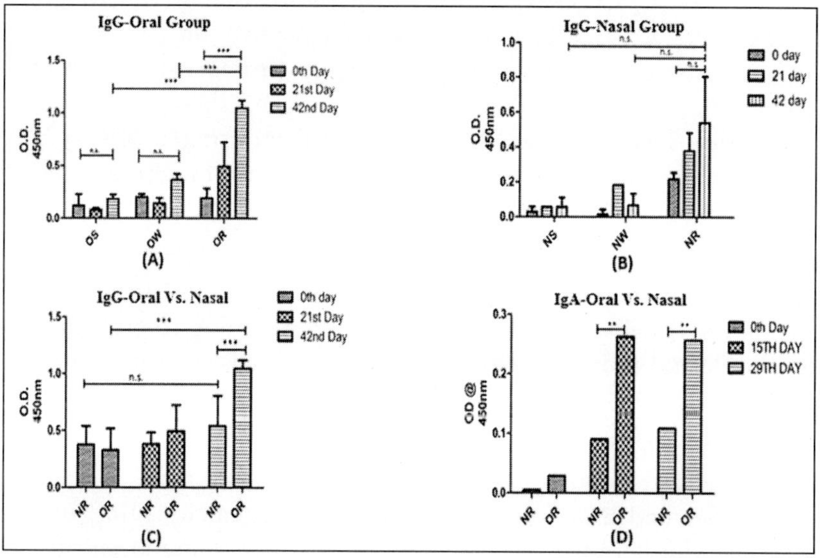

Fig. 3. Anti-OmpA serum IgG and fecal SIgA responses elicited after either oral or nasal administration of r-*L. lactis* expressing OmpA. **(A)** Sera obtained on days 0, 21 and 42 from the group of mice immunized orally with r-*L. lactis* expressing OmpA (OR), wild type *L. lactis* NZ9000 (OW) and saline (OS) were tested for the presence of OmpA specific IgG by ELISA. **(B)** Sera obtained on days 0, 21 and 42 from the group of mice immunized intranasally with r-*L. lactis* expressing OmpA (NR), wild type *L. lactis* NZ9000 (NW) and saline (NS) were tested for the presence of OmpA specific IgG by ELISA. **(C)** Comparative analysis of OmpA specific serum IgG levels in NR and OR group of mice on days 0, 21, and 42. **(D)** Comparative analysis of OmpA specific SIgA levels in fecal samples of OR and NR group on days 0, 15 and 29.

5.2 Exploring Potential of L. Lactis in DNA Delivery

Immunization with plasmid DNA has revolutionized the concept of vaccination. In order to develop a *L. lactis* as DNA delivery platform, a novel DNA vaccine reporter plasmid; pPERDBY was constructed (Yagnik *et al.,* 20017). The functional integrity of pPERDBY was ascertained by detection of EGFP expression at both mRNA and protein levels following transfection of CHO-K1 and Caco-2 cells with the generated construct. The delivery of pPERDBY was achieved by both non-invasive and invasive strains of *L. lactis*, expressing the invasive protein; internalin A of *Listeria monocytogenes*. The comparative FACS analysis revealed threefold increase in the number of EGFP expressing cells in case of the invasive strain as compared to the non-invasive counterpart (Yagnik *et al.*, 2017). Moreover, the present work examined *in vivo* delivery potential of the non-invasive r-*L. lactis*::pPERDBY (*LacVax® DNA-I*) in BALB/c mice. Furthermore, the immune responses elicited by *LacVax® DNA-I* were also characterized and compared with other conventional vaccination approaches, i.e. protein and naked DNA immunization, using EGFP as a model antigen. Presence of antigen specific serum IgG and fecal SIgA antibodies demonstrated *in vivo* DNA delivery and immune stimulating potential of the developed *LacVax® DNA-I* (data in communication).

The present work contributes to the development of putative prophylactic candidates against *Shigella* using the food grade bacteria, *L. lactis* as antigen (Protein/DNA) delivery vehicle. Further studies aiming to evaluate both safety profile and protective efficacy in higher animals are warranted.

6. CONCLUSIONS AND FUTURE PROSPECTS

We have identified immunogenic conserved antigens OmpA, OmpC and their epitopes and also confirmed their immunogenicity using *in silico* approaches. Furthermore, we have confirmed their immunogenicity and protective efficacy using inhouse developed murine shigellosis model. Our main aim is to develop a cross protective oral vaccine, which provides mucosal immunity along with systemic immunity in a safe way against shigellosis. We have successfully engineered food grade *L. lactis* to deliver the OmpA at the mucosal surface *via* the oral route. Developed vaccine candidate *LacVax®:OmpA* successfully stimulates the desired immune responses and protects Balb/C mice against lethal challenge of *S. flexneri*. In addition, we have constructed novel DNA vaccine reporter plasmid pPERDBY which has immunostimulatory CpG motifs and has the capability to replicate in *E. coli* as well as certain strains of *Lactic Acid Bacteria* (LAB). The *in vitro* delivery of pPERDBY to Caco-2 cells was achieved by non-invasive as well as invasive strain of *L. lactis*. The *in vivo* delivery of pPERDBY using noninvasive *L. lactis* (*LacVax® DNA-I*) resulted in humoral and cellular immune responses against a model antigen EGFP in BALB/c mice. Moreover, we have compared for the first time the induced immune response by orally administered *LacVax® DNA-I* with conventional vaccination approaches (Intra mascular delivery of *LacVax® DNA-I and Protein immunization).*

Further work is required to enhance the efficacy of Mucosal epithelium. This can be achieved by optimizing dosage, constitute expression of OmpA, incorporation and targeting the vaccine to Mucosal epithelium (M-cells). It is also essential to perform additional studies to understand the mechanism of immune stimulation which may help in improvising the current vaccine design. Though, the present study deployed food grade *L. lactis* as an antigen delivery vehicle, it is critical to study the safety profile of the engineered recombinant *L. lactis*. The present work established non-invasive as well as invasive *L. lactis* as a DNA delivery vehicle. The immune stimulation following DNA delivery by *L. lactis* against a model antigen EGFP encouraged its application for enteric pathogens wherein EGFP-encoding gene will be replaced by gene encoding potent antigenic protein (for *e.g.* OmpA or OmpC) in pPERDBY. These studies on immune responses following DNA delivery will demonstrate the potential of *L. lactis* as a DNA vaccine delivery candidate. The success of the experiment proposed here may lead to development of an effective vaccine for *Shigella*. Moreover, *L. lactis* based antigen delivery vehicle can be established as a vaccine platform for other infectious diseases.

REFERENCES

[1] Kotloff, K.L., Nataro, J.P., Blackwelder, W.C. *et al.* (2013). Burden and aetiology of diarrhoeal disease in infants and young children in developing countries (the Global Enteric Multicenter Study, GEMS): a prospective, case-control study. *The Lancet* 382: 209–222.

[2] Kotloff, K.L., Riddle, M.S. and Zaidi, A.K.M. (2018). Shigellosis. *The Lancet* 391: 801–812

[3] Levine, M.M., Kotloff, K.L., Barry, E.M. *et al.* (2007). Clinical trials of *Shigella* vaccines: two steps forward and one step back on a long, hard road. *Nat Rev Microbiol.* 5: 540–553.

[4] Mallett, C.P., Van DeVerg, L., Collins, H.H. and Hale, T.L. (1993). Evaluation of *Shigella* vaccine safety and efficacy in an intranasally challenged mouse model. Vaccine 11: 190-196.

[5] Mani, S., Wierzba, T. and Walker, R.I. (2016). Status of vaccine research and development for *Shigella*. *Vaccine* 34: 2887–2894.

[6] Phalipon, A. and Sansonetti, P.J. (2007). Shigella's ways of manipulating the host intestinal innate and adaptive immune system: a tool box for survival? *Immunol Cell Biol.* 85:119-129.

[7] Sansonetti, P.J. (2001). Rupture, invasion and inflammatory destruction of the intestinal barrier by Shigella, making sense of prokaryote-eukaryote cross-talks. *FEMS Microbiol Rev.* 25: 3–14.

[8] Sharma, D. and Padh, H. (2018). Design and development of epitope based vaccine against diarrheal diseases. A Thesis-submitted to Saradar Patel University for the degree of Ph.D. 2018.

[9] Sharma, D., Patel, S., Padh, H. and Desai, P. (2016). Immunoinformatic identification of potential epitopes against *Shigellosis. Intern J of Peptide Research and Therapeutics* 22: 481–495.

[10] Sharma, D., Yagnik, B., Baksi, R., Desai, N., Padh, H. and Desai, P. (2016). Shigellosis murine model established by intraperitoneal and intranasal route of administration: a comparative comprehension overview. *Microbes Infect* 6: 1–8.

[11] Taneja, N. (2007). Changing epidemiology of *Shigellosis* and emergence of Ciprofloxacin-resistant Shigellae in India. *J Clin Microbiol* 45: 678–679.

[12] Turbyfill, K.R., Joseph, S.W. and Oaks, E.V. (1995). Recognition of three epitopic regions on invasion plasmid antigen C by immune sera of Rhesus monkeys infected with *Shigella flexneri* 2a. *Infect Immun.* 63: 3927–3935.

[13] WHO (2006). Shigellosis: State of the art of new vaccine research and development (PDF). Immunization, Vaccines and Biologicals. *World Health Organization* pp. 10–12.

[14] Xia, S., Xu, B., Huang, L., *et al.,* (2011). Prevalence and characterization of human *Shigella* infections in Henan Province, China, in 2006. *J Clin Microbiol* 49: 232–242.

[15] Yagnik, B., Padh, H. and Desai, P. (2016). Construction of a new shuttle vector for DNA delivery into mammalian cells using non-invasive *Lactococcus lactis. Microbes Infect* 18: 237–244.

[16] Yagnik, B., Patel, S., Dave, M., Sharma, D., Padh, H. and Desai, P. (2016). Factors affecting inducible expression of Outer Membrane Protein A (OmpA) of *Shigella dysenteriae* Type-1 in *Lactococcus lactis* using Nisin inducible controlled expression (NICE). *Indian J Microbiol* 56: 80–87.

[17] Yagnik, B., Sharma, D., Padh, H. and Desai, P. (2017). Dual recombinant *Lactococcus lactis* for enhanced delivery of DNA vaccine reporter plasmid pPERDBY. *Microbiol Immunol* 61: 123–129.

[18] Yagnik, B., Sharma, D., Padh, H. and Desai, P. (2017). Immunization with *r-Lactococcus lactis* expressing outer membrane protein A of *Shigella dysenteriae* type-1: evaluation of oral and intranasal route of administration. *J Appl Microbiol* 122: 493–505.

[19] Yang, J.Y., Lee, S.N., Chang, S.Y., *et al.* (2014). A mouse model of shigellosis by intraperitoneal infection. *J Infect Dis.* 209: 203–215.

[20] Zaidi, M.B. and Estrada-García, T. (2014). *Shigella*: A highly virulent and elusive pathogen. *Curr Trop Med Rep* 1: 81–87.

[21] Zhang, W., Luo, Y., Li, J., Lin, L., Ma, Y., Hu, C., Jin, S., Ran, L. and Cui, S. (2011). Wide dissemination of multidrug-resistant *Shigella* isolates in China. *Journal of Antimicrobial Chemotherapy* 66: 2527–2535.

[22] Zhang, Z., Jin, L., Champion, G., Seydel, K.B. and Stanley, Jr., S.L. (2001). *Shigella* infection in a SCID mouse-human intestinal xenograft model: role for neutrophils in containing bacterial dissemination in human intestine. *Infection and Immunity* 69: 3240–3247.

Ten Years of Clinical Research in Novel Investigational Vaccines in Latin America and the Caribbean

Giuliana Oyola-Lozada[1*], Hans Vasquez[2] and Evan Siegel[1, 3]

[1]The University of Queensland, St. Lucia QLD 4072, Brisbane, Australia

[2]Universidad Peruana Cayetano Heredia, Av. Honorio Delgado 430, San Martín de Porres, 15102 Lima, Peru

[3]Ground Zero Pharmaceuticals, 100 Spectrum Center Drive Suite 900 Irvine, CA 92618 California, USA

*E-mail: m.oyolalozada@uq.net.au

ABSTRACT: The number of clinical trials conducted in Latin America and the Caribbean (LAC) has increased in the past few decades due to high disease burden and geographical positioning of the region. However, it is unknown to what extent clinical research is focused on investigational vaccines with significant impact outcome in preventing infectious diseases of high prevalence in LAC. The work is needed to mapping the landscape of clinical research conducted in LAC recently (within 10 years) and consequently assess the development of novel preventive vaccines against infectious agents. A cross-sectional analysis using retrospective data on clinical trials conducted in LAC and registered between 01/01/2008 and 28/02/2018 retrieved from International Clinical Trials Registry Platform (ICTRP). Data retrieved were classified according to categories such as year of registration, country site, target disease, phase of study and type of sponsor. In the 145 studies registered in ICTRP analyzed showed that majority of trials conducted in the last ten years, were late phase studies (III and IV). Vaccines targeting influenza, meningitis, dengue and human papillomavirus were intensively researched. Funding of vaccine clinical studies are mainly by the pharma industry (76.6%), followed by Governmental institutions (17.2%) and Universities (5.5%). Vaccination has been one of the most critical strategies for the control and prevention of infectious diseases affecting large populations in LAC thus clinical research/trials is an imperative in bringing new, effective, safe and high quality vaccines into the market. Renewed efforts are needed to attract the interest of industry, academic or public institutions in investigating new candidate vaccines using modern technologies, primarily to address endemic neglected diseases and emerging and re-emerging infections with high prevalence that has remain under-treated.

Keywords: Clinical Trials, Vaccine Development, LAC, Latin American and the Caribbean Countries, Infectious Diseases.

1. INTRODUCTION

The implementation of the Expanded Programme on Immunization (EPI) of the Americas in 1977 has been the corner stone of major enhancements in health outcomes related to *Vaccine-Preventable Diseases (VPDs)* in Latin America and the Caribbean (LAC) (PAHO, 2015). Due to important efforts deployed by the *Pan American Health Organisation (PAHO)* and the commitment of governments across the region, five VPDs (Smallpox, Poliomyelitis, Rubella and Measles) have been successfully eradicated in the USA to date (PAHO 2016). The introduction of new vaccines has broadly benefitted the LAC population. An important example is the rotavirus vaccine, which after its adoption in some national programmes, has substantially reduced hospitalisation and mortality rates due to diarrhoea in children less than five years of age (Paternina-Caicedo *et al.,* 2015, Santos *et al.,* 2016). In spite of the efforts made so far to implement control strategies against infectious diseases, there are still major implementation concerns in LAC (Barreto *et al.,* 2012). According to the 2016 *Global Burden of Disease Study (GBD)* data, more than 265000 deaths in LAC were attributable to infectious diseases (GBDS 2016). Also, approximately 8% of the total burden of disease is due to *Neglected Tropical Diseases (NTDs)* (*e.g.* Chagas, Dengue, Leishmaniasis and Hookworm infections) (Hotez *et al.,* 2008).

Although vaccines against majority of diseases of global interest have been developed and seems effective however, those designed primarily for use in 2nd and 3rd world endemic settings need either to be effectively developed (Greenwood 2014) or improvements made to their protective immunity or design (Ishikawa *et al.,* 2014). Some infectious diseases prevalent in LAC regions in which vaccines are sought for include, helminths (hookworm, schistosomiasis, trichuriasis, ascariasis, lymphatic filariasis, cysticercosis, onchocerciasis and hydatid diseases like echinococcosis), Protozoa (leishmaniasis and Chagas disease), bacteria (trachoma, leprosy, TB), Virus (dengue, hantavirus, HTLV, yellow fever encephalomyelitis, chikungunya, zika and hepatitis-E). This implies the development of new or improved vaccine candidates that, target specific needs of the region (*i.e.*

covering specific strains circulating in low-income countries and optimising the number of doses needed) (Saul and O'Brien 2017), which will have a large public health impact and alleviate the economic burden of preventable infectious diseases affecting in LAC region (Bacon *et al.,* 2013, Lee *et al.,* 2011; Lee *et al.,* 2010; WHO 2012).

It is obvious that clinical trials are the most important component for the development of novel medicinal products, providing the safety and efficacy of data that will support the marketing authorisation of new drug (Lang and Siribaddana 2012). Generally, pre-licensure clinical evaluation of vaccines comprises three phases: ***Phase-1*** initial testing in a small number of healthy adults; ***Phase-2*** evaluation of safety and preliminary immunogenicity data, and ***Phase-3*** pivotal/confirmatory studies, intended to fully assess the protective efficacy and safety of the new vaccine (WHO 2004). The proportion of clinical trials conducted in industrialized settings (*i.e.* North America and Europe) was considerably higher than those conducted in lower-middle income countries (Thiers *et al.,* 2008), however, over the last few years there has been a growing trend towards the globalisation of clinical trials. The later has been driven by factors such as economics and logistics, harmonisation of international standards for clinical research, improved research infrastructure, institutionalization of regulatory authorities and the imperative to gather data from geographically different sites to support equivalent safety and efficacy across different ethnic groups (Drain *et al.,* 2018, Lang and Siribaddana 2012, Richter 2014, Thiers *et al.,* 2008). Studies of clinical trials registered at *International Clinical Trial Registry Platform (ICTRP)* within the last two decades showed an important growth in the number of trials conducted in lower-middle income settings, especially in Asian and Latin American countries (Drain *et al.,* 2014, Viergever and Li 2015). From 2005 to 2012, trials conducted in Latin American and the Caribbean region have grown at an annual average rate of 12%, whereas other regions showed growth rates less than 8% (Drain *et al.,* 2014). Also, in 2016, approximately 5% of the most popular locations for vaccine trials were countries from Latin America and the Caribbean (Grenham and Villafana 2017). However, the increasing number of human trials might not necessarily be aligned with regional health priorities, such as neglected local diseases including Chagas disease, Dengue and other transmittable diseases (Alger *et al.,* 2009, Da Silva *et al.,* 2017).

This study thus, seeks to review the landscape of clinical trials conducted in LAC region for the development of preventive vaccines against infectious diseases in the last decade, and to assess the gaps between vaccine clinical research in LAC and the pending agenda for vaccine development in the region.

2. MATERIALS AND METHODS

2.1 Study Samples

To analyse the landscape of vaccine clinical trials in LAC region, we employed data for all clinical trials for preventive vaccines conducted in the region that were registered at WHO ICTRP from 01/01/2008 to 28/02/2018. We downloaded these data, examined them, and excluded studies that did not fulfill the inclusion criteria *i.e.* Studies conducted in Non-Latin Caribbean countries, observational studies, duplicate studies, trials conducted for other than prophylactic vaccines (*i.e.* treatment vaccines) or other type of studies in compatible with the aim of this research.

2.2 Data Extraction and Classifications

We extracted the information from registered trials by year of registration, country (ies) site, target disease, Phase of study (I-IV) and type of primary sponsor (Industry, Government, University, non-profit organisation) for each trial retrieved.

2.3 Data Analysis

Descriptive statistical analysis was carried out using Microsoft Excel and summarised to be presented in the tables and graphics.

3. RESULTS

3.1 Registered Clinic Trials

At the time of presentation of this result February 2018, 171 vaccine clinical trials were conducted in LAC and registered at WHO ICTRP and, after excluding results incompatible with the aims of the research, 145 studies were selected for further analysis (see Figure 1). In this search vaccine trials enrolled participants of at least one of these countries: *Argentina*, *Brazil*, *Chile*, *Colombia*, *Mexico*, *Peru*, *Dominican Republic*, *Ecuador*, *Honduras*, *Nicaragua*, *Panama*, *Guatemala*, *Venezuela* and *Costa Rica*.

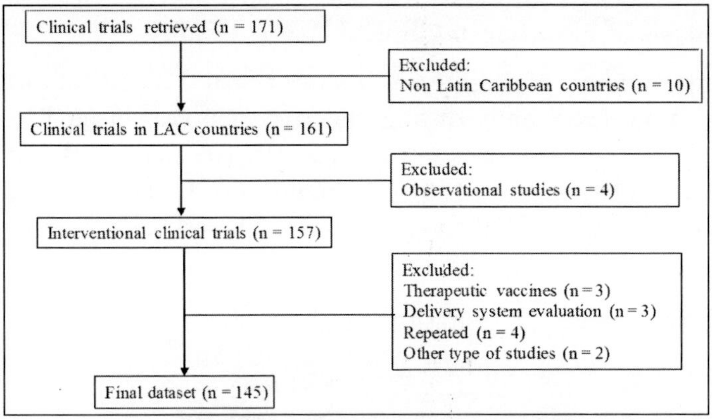

Fig. 1: Flowchart of the Sampling Process of Clinical Trials Registered at ICTRP Included in the Study

3.2 Target Diseases for Vaccine Trials in LAC

The most studied conditions for the development of preventive vaccines were Influenza (22.1%), Meningitis (13.1%), Dengue (12.4%) and HPV (11.7%). Noticeably, there was only one prophylactic vaccine targeting hookworm infection, a soil-transmitted helminthiasis considered a neglected disease highly prevalent in LAC region. Also, one vaccine was found against Zika, an emerging arboviral disease (see Figure 2).

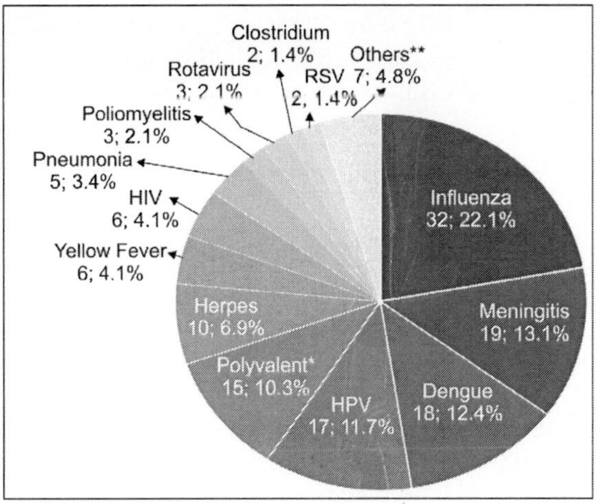

Fig. 2: Target Diseases in Vaccine Trials in LAC Countries (2008–2018)

HPV: Human Papillomavirus; HIV: Human Immunodeficiency Virus; RSV: Respiratory Syncytial Virus.

* Polyvalent vaccines: Measles and Rubella, Infanrix-hexa, Pentavalent DTwP-HepB-Hib, MMR, DTPa-HBV-IPV/Hib, DTaP-IPV-Hep B-PRP-T, DPT.

** Cholera (1), *E.coli* (1), hookworm (1), malaria (1), norovirus (1), chickenpox (1), zika (1).

3.3 Analysis of Number of Clinical Phase Trials

The total number of registered interventional vaccine clinical trials remained almost constant during the past ten years (see Figure 3a). Noticeably, the largest number of studies were late stage studies Phase-III (n = 84) and Phase-IV (n = 10) (see Figure 3b). Only 9 and 28 studies registered at WHO ICTRP corresponded to Phase-I and Phase-II studies, respectively.

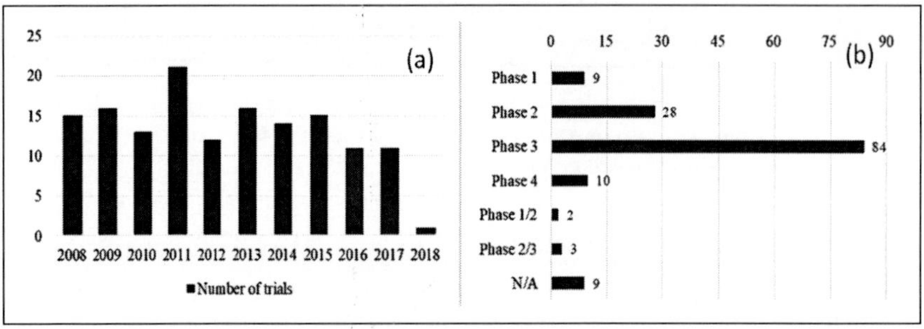

Fig. 3: Number of Clinical Trials for Preventive Vaccines LAC Countries (2008–2010) (a) Year of Registration, (b) Phase of Study of Trials at WHO ICTR, N/A-not Available

3.4 Funding Mechanism

Of the 145 studies, more than 76% were sponsored by industry. Government agencies and Universities sponsored 17.2% and 5.5%, respectively; and only one study (0.7%) had a non-profit organisation as its primary sponsor (see Table 1).

Table 1: Clinical Trials Conducted by Type of Sponsor

Primary Sponsor	*Targeted Vaccines*
Industry (n = 111; 76.6%)	Cholera (1), E. coli (1), HIV(1) Noro virus (1), Chickenpox (1), RSV (2), Clostridium (2), Yellow Fever (2), Poliomyelitis (2), Rotavirus (2), Pneumonia (3), Herpes (10), Polyvalent vaccines (11), Dengue (16), HPV (13), Meningitis (16) Influenza (27)
Government (n = 25; 17.2%)	Malaria (1), Zika (1), Poliomyelitis (1), Rotavirus (1) HIV (3), Pneumonia (1), Yellow fever (3), Polyvalent vaccines (3), Dengue (2), Meningitis (3), HPV (2), Influenza (4)
Universities (n = 8; 5.5%)	Hookworm (1), Pneumonia (1), Yellow fever (1), Polyvalent vaccine (1), HPV (3), influenza (1)
Non-Profit Organisation (n = 1; 0.7%)	HIV (1)

4. DISCUSSIONS

The development of prophylactic vaccines to control major vaccine-preventable infectious diseases may play a crucial role in decreasing morbidity and mortality rates registered in LAC. The results reveal insights of ongoing progress and existing gaps from past clinical development programs for new candidate vaccines conducted across LAC and registered at WHO ICTRP. First, we documented a gap between the target conditions of the investigational products and the diseases that are high priorities for research in vaccine trials. Most of the vaccine candidates evaluated in the region are intended to prevent globally prevalent diseases. Apart from dengue vaccine, which was broadly studied in LAC where the disease is highly endemic (Vannice, Durbin, & Hombach, 2016), only a few trials were designed to evaluate highly prevalent conditions or emerging infections in LAC. The results are consistent with previous studies that found limited trial numbers designed to study local health conditions. Reveiz *et al.,* (2013) found that only 3.8% of published randomised trials conducted in LAC, either for drug development or other interventions, involved study of high priority infectious diseases where only 3.1% of randomised clinical trials evaluated vaccines A similar trend is observed in a recent report of clinical studies registered at WHO ITCRP, where transmissible diseases (*e.g.* HIV, TB, Dengue) and neglected diseases arouse little interest in LAC region (Da Silva *et al.*, 2017). It should be noted that there are a few exceptions to this trend, for example Phase-1 study of Na-GST-1, a candidate vaccine against hookworm disease, which affects approximately 30 million people in the region, was tested by the Sabin Vaccine Institute in Brazilian participants in 2010 (P.J. Hotez *et al.*, 2013; WHO ICTRP, 2010). Also, vaccines against mosquito-borne diseases (Malaria, Yellow Fever and Zika) were assessed in LAC in the last ten years. According to the PAHO, the burden caused by these diseases is alarming thus, between 2015 and 2016, 452,248 cases of Malaria and Yellow Fever was reported in the region (PAHO 2017a). A similar situation has been observed for Zika, which as of August 2017, was found across 48 LAC territories, causing 223,477 autochthonous confirmed cases since 2015 (PAHO 2017b, 2018). Altogether, hookworm, yellow fever, Malaria and Zika vaccine trials made up only 6.2% (n = 9) of the clinical trials registered at WHO ICTRP; therefore, a future direction would be to establish research priorities and to define suitable target product characteristics of new or improved cost-effective vaccines (Saul & O'Brien, 2017).

Another finding is the high numbers of late Phase (3-4) trials and the corresponding low number of Phase-1 and 2 trials conducted in LAC countries. This trend may respond to low pharma R&D levels in the region and low degree of innovation. For instance, the region accounts for less than 0.2% of the total patents in USA in 2012, far from other regions like East Asia that registered more than 30% (Núñez Sellés, 2014). Other than Brazil, no country in Latin America spends more than 1% of Gross Domestic Product (GDP) on R&D and the majority of them spend less than 0.5%, lag behind the average of lower middle-income economies (UNESCO, 2015). Early phase vaccine studies in LAC should be encouraged, for sound scientific and ethical arguments that acknowledge the importance of conducting first in human studies in endemic settings for the target disease (Kapiriri *et al.*, 2011). Also this would strengthen clinical research capacities in the region, which might ultimately, impact population access to safe, high quality, efficacious and affordable vaccines while reducing the dependency on products coming from outside LAC region (Kapiriri *et al.*, 2011; Okpechi, Swanepoel, & Venter, 2015). Furthermore, due to the increasing trend to move Phase-2 and 3 trials to developing countries (Glickman *et al.*, 2009), it is of utmost importance to continue improving clinical research infrastructure, elevate ethical standards and overcome regulatory deficiencies that could discourage conducting early studies in LAC (Grenham & Villafana, 2017). For example, Brazilian Innovation Policy for vaccines is generating important results in the clinical development of novel vaccines for infectious diseases. Brazilian strategy has been focused on strengthening research capacity, investing in infrastructure for clinical research, and providing public support to institutions responsible for clinical trials oversight (Homma *et al.*, 2013).

Our study reveals striking information in the type of primary sponsor of the vaccine studies. Industry sponsors were involved in more than 70% of trials conducted in the region. It has been argued that clinical trials conducted by the industry in Latin America are not aligned with regional disease priorities (Nuria Homedes & Ugalde, 2014). Given this situation, LAC should ensure that industry-sponsored research, put countries and participant's interests ahead of business interests (Núria Homedes & Ugalde, 2016; Ugalde & Homedes, 2014), and this cannot be achieved without the active involvement of LAC governments. Moreover, driving innovation through *Product Development Partnerships (PDPs)* has a key role in advancing vaccines intended to control infectious diseases in LAC (Ho *et al.*, 2011; Huzair, Borda-Rodriguez, & Upton, 2011). Finally, novel technologies, including different vaccine types, adjuvants and immunezation devices, should also be prioritised in the regional research agenda.

5. CONCLUSIONS

Clinical research is of vital in bringing new, effective, safe and quality vaccines into the LAC market. Characterizing clinical trials conducted in the region could assist policymakers in prioritizing strategies and future actions to drive clinical research for the development of new or improved vaccines according to regional interests. Renewed efforts are needed to attract the interest of industry, academia or public institutions to invest in more candidate vaccines using modern technologies, primarily to address endemic high prevalence neglected diseases, emerging and re-emerging infections that are still under-treated in LAC.

REFERENCES

[1] Alger, J., Becerra-Posada, F., Kennedy, A., Martinelli, E., Cuervo, L.G. (2009). National health research systems in Latin America: A 14-country review. *Revista Panamericana de Salud Publica* 26: 447–457.

[2] Bacon, K.M., Hotez, P.J., Kruchten, S.D., Kamhawi, S., Bottazzi, M.E., Valenzuela J.G. Lee B. Y. (2013). The potential economic value of a cutaneous leishmaniasis vaccine in seven endemic countries in the Americas. *Vaccine* 31: 480–486.

[3] Barreto, S.M., Miranda, J.J., Figueroa, J.P., Schmidt, M.I., Munoz, S., Kuri-Morales, P.P., Silva, J.J.B. (2012). Epidemiology in Latin America and the caribbean: Current situation and challenges. *International Journal of Epidemiology* 41: 557–571.

[4] Da Silva, R.E., Amato, A.A., Guilhem, D.B., de Carvalho, M.R., Novaes, M.R.C.G. (2017). International clinical trials in Latin American and caribbean countries: Research and development to meet local health needs. *Frontiers in Pharmacology* 8: 961.

[5] Drain, P.K., Parker, R.A., Robine, M., Holmes, K.K. (2018). Global migration of clinical research during the era of trial registration. *Plos One* 13: e0192413.

[6] Drain, P.K., Robine, M., Holmes, K.K., Bassett, I.V. (2014). Trial watch: Global migration of clinical trials in the era of trial registration. *Nature Reviews Drug discovery* 13: 166–167.

[7] Glickman, S.W., McHutchison, J.G., Peterson, E.D., Cairns, C.B., Harrington, R.A., Califf, R.M., Schulman, K.A. (2009). Ethical and scientific implications of the globalization of clinical research. *N Engl J Med* 360: 816–823.

[8] GBDS (2016). Global burden of disease study 2016 (gbd 2016) results. Retrieved from: https://vizhub.healthdata.org

[9] Greenwood, B. (2014). The contribution of vaccination to global health: Past, present and future. *Philosophical Transactions of the Royal Society B: Biological Sciences* 369: 20130433.

[10] Grenham, A., Villafana, T. (2017). Vaccine development and trials in low and lower-middle income countries: Key issues, advances and future opportunities. *Human Vaccine Immunotherapy* 13: 2192–2199.

[11] Ho, P.L., Miyaji, E.N., Oliveira M.L.S., Dias W.D.O., Kubrusly F.S., Tanizaki M.M., Raw I. (2011). Economical value of vaccines for the developing countries—the case of instituto butantan, a public institution in brazil. *PLOS Neglected Tropical Diseases* 5: e1300.

[12] Homedes, N., Ugalde, A. (2014). Globalization and clinical research in Latin America. In N. Homedes & A. Ugalde (Eds.), Clinical trials in Latin America: Where ethics and business clash (pp. 55–78). Cham: Springer International Publishing.

[13] Homedes, N., Ugalde, A. (2016). Health and ethical consequences of outsourcing pivotal clinical trials to Latin America: A cross-sectional, descriptive study. *Plos One* 11: e0157756.

[14] Homma, A., Tanuri, A., Duarte, A.J., Marques, E., de Almeida, A., Martins, R., Possas, C. (2013). Vaccine research, development, and innovation in Brazil: A translational science perspective. *Vaccine* 31: B54–60.

[15] Hotez P.J., Bottazzi M.E., Franco-Paredes C., Ault S.K., Periago M.R. (2008). The neglected tropical diseases of Latin America and the Caribbean: A review of disease burden and distribution and a roadmap for control and elimination. *PLOS Neglected Tropical Diseases* 2: e300.

[16] Hotez P.J., Diemert D., Bacon K.M., Beaumier C., Bethony J.M., Bottazzi M.E., Russell P. K. (2013). The human hookworm vaccine. Vaccine 31: B227–232.

[17] Huzair F., Borda-Rodriguez A., Upton M. (2011). Twenty-first century vaccinomics innovation systems: Capacity building in the global south and the role of product development partnerships (pdps). *Omics* 15: 539–543.

[18] Ishikawa T., Yamanaka A., Konishi E. (2014). A review of successful flavivirus vaccines and the problems with those flaviviruses for which vaccines are not yet available. *Vaccine* 32: 1326–1337.

[19] Kapiriri L., Lavery J.V., Singer P.A., Mshinda H., Babiuk L., Daar A.S. (2011). The case for conducting first-in-human (phase 0 and phase 1) clinical trials in low and middle income countries. *BMC Public Health* 11: 811–811.

[20] Lang T., Siribaddana S. (2012). Clinical trials have gone global: Is this a good thing? *PLoS Medicine* 9: e1001228.

[21] Lee B.Y., Bacon K.M., Bailey R., Wiringa A.E., Smith K.J. (2011). The potential economic value of a hookworm vaccine. *Vaccine* 29: 1201–1210.

[22] Lee B.Y., Bacon K.M., Connor D.L., Willig A.M., Bailey R.R. (2010). The potential economic value of a *Trypanosoma cruzi* (chagas disease) vaccine in Latin America. *PLOS Neglected Tropical Diseases* 4: e916.

[23] Núñez Sellés A.J. (2014). Pharma R&D in Latin America. *Pharmaceuticals Policy and Law* 16: 267–275.

[24] Okpechi I.G., Swanepoel C.R., Venter F. (2015). Access to medications and conducting clinical trials in lmics. *Nat Rev Nephrol* 11: 189–194.

[25] PAHO (2015). Pan American Health Organization plan of action on immunisation. In 54th Directing Council of PAHO, 67th session of the regional committee of WHO for the America (Vol. 2018). Washington, D.C., USA.

[26] PAHO (2016). Region of the Americas is declared free of measles. Pan American Health Organization, In (Vol. 2018). Immunization Newsletter.

[27] PAHO (2017a). Health situation in the Americas: Core indicators 2017. Retrieved from http://iris.paho.org/xmlui/bitstream/handle/123456789/34329/CoreIndicators2017_eng.pdf?sequence=1&isAllowed=y (accessed 18 Mar 2017).

[28] PAHO (2017b). Regional zika epidemiological update (Americas). Retrieved from https://www.paho.org/hq/index.php?option=com_content&view=article&id=11599%3Aregional-zika-epidemiological-update-americas&catid=8424%3Acontents&Itemid=41691&lang=fr (accessed 25 Aug 2017).

[29] PAHO (2018). Zika cases and congenital syndrome associated with zika virus reported by countries and territories in the Americas, 2015–2018 cumulative cases. Retrieved from http://www.paho.org/hq/index.php?option=com_docman&task=doc_view&Itemid=270&gid=43296&lang=en (accessed 15 Jun 2017).

[30] Paternina-Caicedo A., Parashar U.D., Alvis-Guzmán N., De Oliveira L.H., Castaño-Zuluaga A., Cotes-Cantillo K. De la Hoz-Restrepo F. (2015). Effect of rotavirus vaccine on childhood diarrhea mortality in five Latin American countries. *Vaccine* 33: 3923–3928.

[31] Reveiz L., Sangalang S., Glujovsky D., Pinzon C.E., Asenjo Lobos C., Cortes M., Bonfill X. (2013). Characteristics of randomized trials published in Latin America and the Caribbean according to funding source. *Plos One* 8: e56410.

[32] Richter T.A. (2014). Clinical Research: A globalized network. *Plos One* 9: e115063.

[33] Santos V.S., Marques D.P., Martins-Filho P.R.S., Cuevas L.E., Gurgel R.Q. (2016). Effectiveness of rotavirus vaccines against rotavirus infection and hospitalization in Latin America: Systematic review and meta-analysis. *Infectious Diseases of Poverty* 5: 83.

[34] Saul A., O'Brien K.L. (2017). Prioritizing vaccines for developing world diseases. *Vaccine* 35: A16–A19.

[35] Thiers F.A., Sinskey A.J., Berndt E.R. (2008). Trends in the globalization of clinical trials. *Nature Reviews Drug Discovery* 7: 13.

[36] Ugalde A., Homedes N. (2014). Conclusion. In N. Homedes & A. Ugalde (Eds.), Clinical trials in Latin America: Where ethics and business clash (pp. 275–282). Cham: Springer International Publishing.

[37] UNESCO (2015). Unesco Science Report: Towards 2030. Retrieved from https://en.unesco.org/unesco_science_report

[38] Vannice K.S., Durbin A., Hombach J. (2016). Status of vaccine research and development of vaccines for dengue. *Vaccine* 34: 2934–2938.

[39] Viergever R.F., Li K. (2015). Trends in global clinical trial registration: An analysis of numbers of registered clinical trials in different parts of the world from 2004 to 2013. *BMJ Open* 5: e008932.

[40] WHO-ICTRP (2010). Safety and immunogenicity of a human hookworm candidate vaccine with or without additional adjuvant in Brazilian adults. Retrieved from http://apps.who.int/trialsearch/Trial2.aspx?TrialID=NCT01261130

[41] WHO (2012). World Health Organisation-Global vaccine action plan 2011–2020: In D.o.V. Collaboration (Ed.).

[42] WHO (2004). Expert Committee on Biological Standardization. Guidelines on clinical evaluation of vaccines: Regulatory expectations. In Fifty-Second Report. Annex 1. Geneva.

Bioinformatics-Based Approach as a Novel Platform to Identify Putative Therapeutic Drug Targets and Vaccine Candidates for Plasmodium vivax

Abraham Isah*[1], Abdulrazak B. Ibrahim[1] and Kindzeka Lesley[2]

[1]Department of Biochemistry, Faculty of Life Sciences,
Ahmadu Bello University, Zaria, Nigeria

[2]Department of Biochemistry, Faculty of Sciences,
Usmanu Danfodiyo University, Sokoto, Nigeria

*E-mail: abraham2637@gmail.com

ABSTRACT: Plasmodium (p) vivax ranks second prevalent cause of malaria and has the widest geographical distribution around the globe. Lack of vaccine candidates is the paramount reason why malaria still remains a public health problem. The need to search for new vaccine candidates is very urgent as no vaccine against malaria has been certified to the date. In the present study a bioinformatics-based approach (vaccine informatics) has been identified as a novel platform to identify drug targets and vaccine candidates for P. vivax. Using subtractive genomic approach, a total of 88536 protein coding sequences of P. vivax were screened for non-human homologous outer membrane proteins. The BLASTp tool of the NCBI database was used for the alignment search. Subcellular localization prediction, outer membrane analysis and membrane topology were analyzed using the PSORTb V.3, vaxijen v2.0 and TMHMM V2 softwares, respectively. B-cell epitopes were predicted using the AAP and BCpred prediction tools. BLASTP similarity search of all enzymes resulted in non homologues enzymes of P. vivax. Plasmodium vivax Sal-1 (XP_001613073.1 and XP_001613073.1) showed the highest vaxijens core of all screened proteins and therefore were suspected the most probable protein to induce both B- and T-cell mediated immunity. The results of the PSORTb server for identification of non-homologous outer membrane proteins showed that the B-cell epitope, GGSGDSGDSGGGRDRGNRSD, is the most probable antigen to serve as a vaccine candidate, while, the three epitopes MSERNSWVRRKIELINSGYK, GRGRPDERDKPDGPKEDSLW and

GIFASQNKELIFTPVLRDGQ can never serve as vaccine candidates. Three membrane associated putative proteins were finally selected based on their exomembrane topology, vaxijen score, TMHMM analysis and IC50 to identify epitopes that can induce both B- and T-cell mediated immunity. They may therefore represent good vaccine candidates subject for further evaluation.

Keywords: Plamodium vivax, Bioinformatics, Epitopes, Vaccine, Topology, Antigen, Homology.

1. INTRODUCTION

One of the most serious health problems worldwide is malaria (Narain 2008). Among 2.6b people at risk of malaria infection, annual estimates of *P. vivax* cases range from 130 to 435 million (Guerra *et al.*, 2005). Lack of vaccine candidates/new targets (Timta 2013) and continuous rising cases of drug/insecticide resistance among malaria parasites and mosquito vectors, respectively (Miller *et al.*, 2013, Timta 2013) are the paramount reasons why malaria still remains a significant public health problem worldwide. *Plasmodium vivax* ranks as the second prevalent cause of malaria after *P. falciparum* (Mohapatra *et al.*, 2008, Carlton *et al.*, 2008) and has the widest geographical distribution around the globe (Eesha 2015, Carlton *et al.*, 2008). Though it seldom causes death, it can still cause severe illness (Eesha 2015). While there are positive effects of vaccination on public health with regards to the global campaign for eradication of smallpox (Yongqun *et al.*, 2010) none has been recorded yet for malaria. Peptide-based sub-unit vaccine were recently been reported to be useful for treating both infectious diseases and cancers (Prabhavathy *et al.*, 2011). The need to search for new targets or vaccine candidates is very urgent (Ajao *et al.*, 2014) as no vaccines against malaria have been certified till date (WHO, 2013). Bioinformatics-based approach (Vaccine informatics) is a novel platform to identify both drug targets and vaccines candidates for *P. vivax* (Yongqun *et al.*, 2010, Ajao *et al.*, 2014). The use of bioinformatics tools in the field of vaccinology has tremendously triggered initiating the potential to revolutionize every aspect of the pre- and post-licensure vaccine enterprise (Yongqun *et al.*, 2010).

Recent availability of comprehensive genomic, transcriptomic and proteomic datasets of pathogens offers tremendous insight for *in silico* information mining (Tomar and De 2010) for prediction of putative therapeutic drug targets and vaccine candidates. Therefore, this study aimed at identifying putative druggable targets and vaccines candidates for *Plasmodium vivax* using bioinformatics tools.

2. MATERIALS AND METHODS

2.1 Protein Sequences Retrieval

A systematic workflow was defined based on the immune-informatics approach for the identification of potential vaccine candidates against *P. vivax* (Sandeep and Rajani 2017) and was modified to suit the aim of this current study. The complete protein of *P. vivax* was downloaded from National Centre for Biotechnology Information (NCBI) server www.nchi.nlm.nih.gov/genomes. A total of 88536 coding sequences was screened. Only coding sequences with 3000 amino acids and above were included.

2.2 Alignment Search

The BLASTp tool of the NCBI database was used (Altshul *et al.,* 1997). Search against the non-redundant database with maximum identity score (MIS) of > 35% as recommended by WHO/FAO (Ping *et al.,* 2015) was done. The e-value cut-off was set at 1.00. The sequence alignment analysis was limited to amino acid sequences from Homo sapiens. One of the exclusion criteria was amino acid sequences homologue to humans. Searches with "NO HIT FOUND" were recorded as "non-human homologous coding sequences" and listed out as putative therapeutic drug target in *P. vivax.* These non-homologous sequences were subjected to BLASTp analysis against the *H. sapiens* at a MIS of > 35% (Ping *et al.,* 2015) and e-value cut off 1.00 (Altshul *et al.,* 1997).

2.3 Sub-cellular Localization Prediction

Sub-cellular localization analysis (Gardy *et al.,* 2005) was carried out using the PSORTb v.3 tool. Only proteins that were not homologous to humans (non-human homologues proteins) were subjected to analysis using this tool.

2.4 Membrane Analysis

Further analyses of all the outer membrane proteins were done using the Vaxijen v.2.0 antigen prediction server. The antigenicity of each full length amino acid sequence was analyzed using a threshold of 0.4 ACC output.

2.5 B-cell Epitope Prediction

Both the BCpreds analysis and the AAP tool were used to identify the B-cell epitopes (NMCP 2007, Chen *et al.,* 2007). For identification of common B-cell epitopes, the prediction only proteins antigenic score of > 0.6 were selected for this analysis. All B-cell epitopes (20mers) having a BCpreds cut off score = 1.0 were selected for further analysis.

2.6 Membrane Topology

The topology of the membrane of selected B-cell epitopes were subsequently checked for exo-membrane amino acid sequences using the TMHMM V 2 tool. MHC classes 1 and 2 epitopes were selected and calculated using the MHCPred V.2 (Guan *et al.,* 2003) selecting [DRB 1*0101] and the Vaxijen tool respectively. Epitopes with IC_{50} less than 50 nM and highest antigenicity value were finally selected.

3. RESULTS

BLASTP similarity search of all enzymes at a MIS of > 35% and e-value cutoff at 1.0 resulted in identifying non-homologues enzymes of *P. vivax* (see Table 1). The higher the Vaxijen score more likely the protein, as

Table 1: Selected *P. vivax* Membrane Associated Non-Human Homologous Protein

Protein	*ID No.*	*Protein Size*	*Vaxijen Score*	*Localisation*	*Inference*
Conserved Plasmodium Membrane Protein	SCO 65189.1	4998	0.6670	Outer membrane	Probable
	SCO 65213.1	3111	0.7464	Cytoplasm	Highly probable
	SCO 65263.1	3703	0.5659	Inner membrane	Not probable
	SCO 65277.1	4127	0.7056	Outer membrane	Highly probable
	SCO 65628.1	3735	0.7223	Outer membrane	Highly probable
	SCO 64898.1	3459	0.7775	Outer membrane	Highly probable
	SCO 64896.1	4034	0.6702	Cytoplasm	Probable
Plasmodium vivax Sal-1	XP_001617138.1	3027	-	Inner	Not an option
	XP_001617147.1	3556	0.8110	Outer membrane	Most probable
	XP_001613409.1	3002	0.5948	Outer membrane	Probable
	XP_001616850.1	4108	0.7104	Cytoplasm	Highly probable
	XP_001613073.1	3695	0.8771	Cytoplasm	Mostly probable
	XP_001613077.1	3680	0.6878	Cytoplasm	Probable
	XP_001616773.1	3546	0.6555	Outer membrane	Probable
Hypothetical Protein	XP_001613100.1	3759	0.8479	Outer membrane	Highly probable
	XP_001613220.1	4648	0.6870	Outer membrane	Probable

a good vaccine candidate *P. vivax* Sal-1 (XP_001613073.1 and XP_001613073.1) showed the highest Vaxijen score of all the screened *P. vivax* proteins and therefore were tagged the most probable protein to induce both B and T-cell mediated immunity.

The result of the PSORTb server identification of non-homologous proteins that resides in the outer membrane resulted in identifying some of the listed proteins in Table 2. Epitopes with the highest AAP/BCpred Score (=1.0) were predicted to induce B and T-cell mediated immunity (see Table 2). The B-cell epitope: GGSGDSGDSGGGRDRGNRSD was identified as the most probable antigen to serve as a vaccine candidate, whereas the three epitopes: MSERNSWVRRKIELINSGYK, GRGRPDE RDKPDGPKEDSLW and GIFASQNKELIFTPVLRDGQ can never serve as vaccine candidates.

Table 2: Selected B-Cell Epitopes Using the BCpreds Tool and Antigenicity of Protein Using the Vaxijen Score

Protein	*Amino Acid Locus*	*B-Cell Epitopes*	*AAP/ BCpred*	*Vaxijen Score*	*Inference*
Plasmodium vivax Sal-1	1414	ISDPSGNGIDGAGKKKYVRR	1	1.6068	Antigen
	1474	SRRSKKNGETGDIYMGIPDP	1	1.3727	Antigen
	293	SESSGGSGSGEKGQNVEYAA	1	2.7443	Antigen
	1077	GIFASQNKELIFTPVLRDGQ	1	-0.2366	Non Antigen
	861	HSVENVNMSSTNGRSDKGSN	1	2.0633	Antigen
Hypothetical protein Plasmodium vivax Sal-1	1177	GGSGDSGDSGGGRDRGNRSD	1	3.0621	Antigen
	740	RNRERKRRNSPSDTASSGCS	1	1.5849	Antigen
	1004	GDSREVHRKAVKNRTGKGAD	1	1.9067	Antigen
	657	VVGGDKGASVGEGKKDSLPG	1	1.4031	Antigen
	2440	QEGGSQEEDPTEENPTEEDP	1	1.6032	Antigen
	3129	MSERNSWVRRKIELINSGYK	1	–0.0226	Non Antigen
	2043	GRGRPDERDKPDGPKEDSLW	1	0.3237	Non Antigen

Table 3: Epitopes Predicted to Induce Both B and T-Cell Mediated Immunity

*Epitopes $MHCP_{red}$ DRBI*0401*	*A/A Position*	*Vaxijen Score*	*Predicted IC_{50} Value (nM)*	*Prediction Confidence (Max = 1)*
GGRDRGNRS	1177	1.0984	44.57	0.78
VNMSSTNGR	861	2.5315	6.016	0.89
KGASGEGEV	426	3.0455	2546.83	1.00

Three membrane associated putative proteins were finally selected based on their exo-membrane topology, vaxijen score, TMHMM analysis and IC_{50} as epitopes that can induce both B and T-cell mediated immunity and hence as potential vaccine candidates (see Table 3).

4. DISCUSSIONS

Similar studies carried out by Aajo *et al.* (2014) on *P. falciparum* predicted three major epitopes by pharmaco-proteomic and genomic sequences studies of *P. vivax*. In this present work, genomic sequences of *P. vivax* were used. T- or B-cell epitopes have previously identified by Menakha *et al.* (2011), Sollner *et al.* (2008) and Arevalo *et al.* (2002). The scientific fact that B- and T-cell inducing epitopes are good targets for designing peptide based vaccines has also been established (Ajao *et al.,* 2014). A definite homology between the host and pathogen protein chosen as drug targets might lead to unwanted cross-reactions and cytotoxicity due to homology between the host and pathogen and was prevented by screening out human homologous sequences Neema *et al.* (2011). Further analysis of non-human homologous proteins in *P. vivax* was carried out for localization in the outer membrane. Prediction of the two selected membrane associated hypothetical proteins were centered on exo-membrane topology and Vaxijen score since epitopes with both B and T-cell mediated immunity property are good vaccine candidates (WHO 2013, Singh and Raghava 2001). Based on the IC_{50}, GGRDRGNRS and VNMSSTNGR were predicted to be good binders with higher affinity (see Table 3). While these two epitopes may therefore be considered as good vaccine candidates, KGASGEGEV epitope is not due to its high IC_{50} (see Table 3).

5. CONCLUSIONS

This work identified GGRDRGNRS and VNMSSTNGR epitopes as good vaccine candidates for P. vivax due to their lower IC_{50} (≤ 50) and their good Vaxijen scores of 1.0984 and 3.0455, respectively. This also means that the two predicted epitopes will have the ability to induce both B and T-cell mediated immune responses thereby eliciting both humoral and cell mediated immunity needed for protection against infection.

REFERENCES

[1] Ajao, A.T., Adekeye, A.O. and Yakubu, S.E. (2014). Application of reverse vaccinology in designing a vaccine for malaria. *American Journal of Bioinformatics Research* 4: 6–10.

[2] Altshul, S.F., Thomas, L.M., Alejandro, A.S., Jinghu, Z. and Zheng, Z. (1997). Gapped BLAST and PSI BLAST; a new generation of protein database search programs. *Nucleic Acids Res* 17: 3389–3402.

[3] Arevalo-Herrea, M., Valencia, A.Z., Vergara, J., Bonelo, A. and Fleischhauer, K. (2002). Identification of HLA-A2 restricted $CD^{8(+)}$ T-lymphocyte responses to *Plasmodium vivax* circum sporozoite protein in individuals naturally exposed to malaria. *Parasite Immunol* 24: 161–169.

[4] Carlton, J.M., Adams, J.H., Silva, J.C. and Fraser-Liggett C.M. (2008). Comparative genomics of the neglected human malaria parasite *Plasmodium vivax. Nature* 455: 757–763.

[5] Chen, J., Liu, H., Yang, J. and Chous, K.C. (2007). Prediction of Linear B-cell epitopes using amino acid pair antigenicity scale. *Amino Acids* 33: 423–428.

[6] Eesha, D (2015). Types of Malaria. Onlymyhealth. http://www.onlymyhealth .com/what-types-malaria-1302068689 (accessed 14th April 2018).

[7] FMOH (2007). National frame work for monitoring and Evaluation of malaria control in Nigeria. Federal Ministry of Health, Abuja, Nigeria.

[8] Gardy, J.L., Laird, M.R. and Chen, F. (2005). PSORTb v.2.0: Expanded prediction of bacterial protein subcellular localization and insights gained from comparative proteome analysis. *Bioinformatics* 21: 617–623.

[9] Guerra, C.A., Snow, R.W. and Hay, S.I. (2005). Mapping the global extent of malaria in 2005. *Trends Parasitol* 22: 353–358.

[10] https://engagedscholarship.csuohio.edu/etdarchive/810.

[11] Menakha, M. and Manoharan, C. (2011). Computer aided drug from immune informatics to reverse vaccinology. *Advanced Biotech* 10: 1444–147.

[12] Miller, L.H., Ackerman, H.C., Su, X.Z. and Wellems, T.E. (2013). Malaria biology and disease pathogene-sis: Insights for new treatments. *Nat Med* 19: 156–167.

[13] Mohapatra, P.K., Prakash, A., Bhattacharyya, D.R., Goswami, B.K., Ahmed, A., Sarmah, B. and Mohant, A.J. (2008). Detection and Molecular confirmation of a focus of *Plasmodium malariae* in Arunachal Pradesh. *Indian J Med Res.* 128: 52–56.

[14] Narain, J.P. (2008). Malaria in the South-East Region: myth and the reality. *Indian J Med Res* 128: 1–3.

[15] Neema, M., Karunasagar, I. and Karunsagar, I. (2011). *In-silico* identification and characterization of novel drug targets and outer membrane proteins in the fish pathogen *Edwards illatarda. Bioinformatics* 3: 37–42.

[16] NMCP (2007). National Malaria Control Programme, Federal Ministry of Heath Annual report Abuja, Nigeria.

[17] Panda, S.K. and Mahapatra, R.K. (2017). *In-silico* screening, identification and validation of a novel vaccine candidate in the fight against *Plasmodium falciparum*. Parasitol Res 116: 1293–1305.

[18] Ping, S., Rod, H. and Siva, K. (2015). Using the power of e-values in FASTA to detect potential allergen cross-reactivity. *Toxicology Reports* 2: 1145–1148.

[19] Prabhavathy, K., Perumal, P. and Sundara, B.N. (2011). *In-silico* identification of B- and T-cell epitopes on OMPLA and LsC from *Salmonella typhi* for peptide-based subunit vaccine design. *Indian Journal of Biotechnology* 10: 440–451.

[20] Singh, H. and Raghava, G.P. (2001). Prediction of HLA-DR binding site. *Bioinformatics* 17: 1238–1237.

[21] Sollner, J., Grohmann, R., Rapberger, R., Perco, P., Lukas, A. and Mayer, B. (2008). Analysis and prediction of protective continuous B-cell epitopes on pathogen proteins. *Immunome Res* 7: 4.

[22] Timta, M.Z. (2013). Bioinformatic Analysis and in Vitro Expression of Malaria Parasite Translocon and Ribonuclease Binding-Like Rhoptry Genes. ETD Archive. 810.

[23] Tomar, N. and De, R.K. (2010). Immuno informatics: an integrated scenario. *Immunology* 131: 153–156.

[24] He, Y, Rino, R., De Groot, A.S. and Chen, R.T. (2010). Vaccine informatics Journal of Biomedicine and Biotechnology. Vol. 2010, Article ID 765762, 2 pages.

An Overview on Schistosomiasis Infection among Nigeria School Age Children and Progress of Vaccine Development

E.O. Ibeh[1]*, I.C.J. Omalu[2], B.O. Ibeh[3], K.A. Adeniyi[2] and P.O. Oko[1]

[1]Department of Biological Sciences, Veritas University Abuja (The Catholic University of Nigeria), Nigeria

[2]Department of Biological Sciences, Federal University of Technology, Minna, Nigeria

[3]Medical Biotechnology, National Biotechnology Development Agency, Abuja, Nigeria

*E-mail: emmanuelaibeh@gmail.com

ABSTRACT: In terms of endemicity, public health and socio-economic burden, schistosomiasis remains one of the most widespread human parasitic diseases and is ranked second after malaria, especially in the Sub-Sahara Africa. Despite the worldwide success of chemotherapy, the disease continues to defy control efforts. The disease is endemic in 78 countries, infecting about 240 million people worldwide and more than 700 million people live under risk in endemic areas. Within Sub-Sahara Africa, Nigeria carries the heaviest burden with an estimated 29 million cases of infection. School children have been identified as the major victim of the disease and transmission is chiefly by the planorbid fresh water snails commonly found around sources of water such as streams, rivers, ponds and irrigation canals. A study carried out in Oyo, for instance, revealed a high (71.4%) prevalence of schistosomiasis among school age children. The burden of schistosomiasis was high among children of migrant workers and they serve as reservoirs for transmission of the disease. Praziquantel, the only drug currently available for treatment, is unable to kill developing schistosomes, it does not prevent re-infection and its continued extensive use may result in the future emergence of drug-resistant parasites. As a result, vaccine strategies represent an essential component as an adjunct to chemotherapy for the future control of schistosomiasis. Vaccination against schistosomes can either target prevention of infection and/or reduction of parasite fecundity. A reduction in worm numbers is the "gold standard" for anti-schistosome vaccine development, with the migrating schistosomulum stage likely to be the major vaccine target of protective immune responses. Over 100 schistosome candidate vaccine antigens have been identified, however, only three molecules, S. mansoni fatty acid binding protein (Sm14), S. mansoni tetraspanin (Sm-TSP-2) and S. haematobium glutathione S-transferase (Sh28GST), have entered human clinical trials. Schistosomes use fatty acid binding proteins (FABPs) to absorb, transport and compartmentalize fatty acids from the host and, because of this critical biological function, Sm14 has long been considered a potential vaccine candidate. Recombinant Sm14 (rSm14) provided up to 67% protection in terms of reduced S. mansoni worm burden in outbred Swiss mice without use of an adjuvant. Sh28GST, a 28 kDa glutathione S-transferase enzyme plays a role in fatty acid metabolism, prostaglandin D2 synthesis and may help the parasite to evade the host immune system. The enzyme present in S. mansoni (Sm28GST) has been tested extensively as a recombinant protein vaccine in various experimental models and has shown partial protection in terms of reduced worm burden, inhibition of female worm fecundity and reduction in egg viability. Sm-p80 Calpain is a calcium activated neutral cysteine protease. Prime-boost vaccination with Sm-p80, the large subunit of S. mansoni calpain, in combination with resiquimod adjuvant, resulted in 49% worm burden reduction, while 50% protection was achieved using the recombinant protein as primary and boost vaccine in mice. Vaccinomics is a powerful innovation which provides a foundation for searching critical determinants of immunity. It can promote both antigen discovery and design of novel vaccines for multi-cellular pathogens such as schistosomes. A recent vaccinomics approach for discovering novel schistosome antigens that may not be revealed by conventional proteomics involved both design and manufacture of an immunomics protein array, the first to be generated for a multi-cellular pathogen. This vaccine could be administered to children between the age of 3 and 12 years to prevent severe infection particularly in high risk population. This review summarizes the state of the art of schistosomiasis vaccine development.

Keywords: Schistosomiasis, Schistosoma Mansoni, S. Japonicum, Immune Response, Vaccine, Antigen Discovery.

1. INTRODUCTION

Schistosomiasis is a Neglected Tropical Diseases (NTDs) caused by parasitic worms of the genus *Schistosoma*. In terms of public health and socio-economic burden, Schistosomiasis remains one of the most widespread human parasitic diseases and ranked second after malaria, especially in the Sub-Sahara Africa (WHO 2016a). The disease is endemic in 78 developing countries, infecting almost 240 million people world-wide, and more than 700 million people live under risk in the endemic areas. Twenty millions of these suffer severe consequences of the disease, 120 million are symptomatic and the rest are usually asymptomatic (Capron *et al.,* 2002, WHO 2016a). Estimates in 2014 showed that at least 258 million people required preventive treatment for Schistosomiasis. Ninety percent of those live in Africa (WHO 2016b). In Africa, Schistosomiasis is endemic in most rural settlement aligning coastal bodies. This is attributed to suitable environmental condition that favours proliferation of the intermediate host (planorbid snails); including river, creek, ponds, lakes and slow flowing water. This water is typically used for domestic activities and indiscriminate sewage disposal (Nwosu *et al.,* 2015). In Africa where the greatest prevalence of infection occurs, it has been estimated that 150,000 people die each year due to Schistosomiasis-related causes (WHO 2011). In Nigeria, one of the most severely affected countries in Africa, it is estimated that 101.28 million people are at risk of infection while 25.83 million are infected. A recent review by Angaye (2016) showed that Schistosomiasis occurs in all the states of the federation.

Schistosomiasis leads to a chronic and debilitating ill health (Enersen 2015, Uneke *et al.,* 2010). The estimates for morbidity in affected populations are high especially among school children between the ages of 6-15 years; children who swim and play in nearby lakes and irrigation channels, women who carryout household chores like fetching water, washing clothes and cooking utensils, fishermen and irrigation workers who always make contact with water for leisure, recreation or as a result of their profession expose themselves to the shedding freely swimming infective larvae of the parasite from the intermediate snail hosts (Okoli and Odaibo 1999, WHO 2010). School age children who live in areas with water bodies that harbour the vectors are most susceptible to the diseases (Okpala 2010, FMOH 2015). Urogenital Schistosomiasis is caused by *Schistosoma haematobium* and whereas intestinal Schistosomiasis is due to infection by *S. mansoni, S. japonicum, S. intercalatum* and S. *mekongi* (WHO 2016b).

Schistosomiasis is a major public health problem in Nigeria but has received little attention. Reasons for the significant burden of the disease includes: poverty, poor environmental sanitation and water supply and poor access to health care facilities. These communities are also hard to reach and therefore underserved by policies and programs aimed at controlling Schistosomiasis and other NTDs (Hotez *et al.,* 2007). There has been no sustained decrease in the prevalence of disease as the prevention, control and treatment programs in Nigeria have been suboptimal (WHO 2010). In 2013, more than 60 million people required treatment for Schistosomiasis, however, treatment programs were available for only a few of the affected population (CIA 2015). The Carter Center along with other development and implementation partners work with the Federal Ministry of Health (FMOH) in Nigeria to treat school age children in priority states for the disease; however these control programmes are yet to have a noticeable effect on the prevalence of Schistosomiasis therefore raising doubts if control can be achieved (SU 2015). Human treatment with PZQ plays a central role in the control and prevention of Schistosomiasis, being the only effective drug currently available (Joseph *et al.,* 2010). However, the drug does not prevent re-infection and its exclusive use for the prevention and control of Schistosomiasis is problematic; having been used for more than three decades, the emergence of PZQ-resistant schistosomiasis a constant threat (Tebeje *et al.,* 2016). Other drawbacks of PZQ are its poor activity against immature schistosomes, resulting in sub-optimal outcomes during mass drug administration campaigns and, as its mechanism of action remains unclear, the design of alternative drug formulations has proven difficult (Cioli *et al.,* 2014). The commonly used molluscicide 'Niclosamide' is effective but to be able to achieve best results; the application has to be done at least twice a year. This is not affordable by the local communities (Oketch *et al.,* 1998). According to WHO (1965), Niclosamide is highly toxic to snails and eggs but difficult to formulate thereby requiring expertise before use. This compound is harmful to non-target organisms like the fish, non-biodegradable, not eco-friendly and there is probability that some resistance to niclosamide can be induced under extreme conditions of genetic selection of the snails (Sulivan *et al.,* 1984). In order to control and finally eliminate Schistosomiasis, a vaccine will likely be a key component of an integrated approach (*i.e.* involving mass chemotherapy, targeted molluscicides, environmental modification, health education, and improved sanitation and vaccination (Tebeje *et al.,* 2016). A transmission blocking vaccine for use in bovines could serve as a vital component in the control of *S. japonicum* (Ross *et al.,* 2013), whereas clinical vaccines against *S. mansoni* and *S. haematobium* need to be developed.

This review evaluates the prevalence of Schistosomiasis among school age children and the current status of schistosome vaccine development. Although complexity of the schistosome life-cycle with its various stages each expressing distinct antigens development, it provides a vehicle for identifying many alternative candidate molecules for vaccine development. The fact that different parasite stages reside in different host niches (larvae in the skin and lungs, adults in the liver and intestine or bladder capillaries) can help in designing potential vaccines to prevent the migration of schistosome parasites and their maturation to adult worms. Importantly, the fact that schistosomes do not replicate in the definitive host makes partial reduction of the parasite burden sufficient to control Schistosomiasis, strengthening the argument for developing an effective vaccine as a control intervention (Hewitson *et al.,* 2014). When identifying a suitable vaccine candidate, it is prudent to select key schistosome molecules in the live parasite that are (a) exposed to the host immune system and (b) are essential for parasite survival. Such components may, for example, function in migration, immune evasion, nutrient uptake or attachment (Tebeje *et al.,* 2016). Adjuvant selection and mode of vaccine formulation and delivery are other important considerations in vaccine design and deployment as they can have a considerable impact on the protective effectiveness of the vaccine. It is well known that, in contrast to attenuated cercarial vaccines, other types, such as subunit vaccines, require an appropriate adjuvant to help stimulating the immune system. A number of adjuvants are available such as gels, emulsions, particulates, cytokines, microbial products (*e.g.* CpG, cholera toxin) and proteases. Adjuvants can overcome immune senescence in older individuals, prolong the immunelogical memory of a vaccine broaden the antibody repertoire and direct the immune system to a Th1 biased, Th2 biased or mixed Th1/Th2 responses (Knudsen *et al.,* 2016). For example, a Th1 driving adjuvant such as IL-12, administered with irradiated cercariae, provided up to 90% protection in murine Schistosomiasis (Lebens *et al.,* 2004, Stephenson *et al.,* 2014). Currently, in order to increase the protective efficacy of schistosome vaccines, a strategy of combining existing adjuvants with novel ones, developed based on emerging immunological targets, has been muted (Stephenson *et al.,* 2014). Some of the other challenges in Schistosomiasis vaccine development are the risk of an atopic IgE response to a candidate vaccine (Diemert *et al.,* 2012), a lack in understanding the nature of the immune response and the correlates of protective immunity in humans and other mammalian hosts, the transmission of other pathogens in Schistosomiasis endemic areas resulting in co-infected individuals which can impact on vaccine efficacy, and antigenic polymorphism (Mo *et al.,* 2014). Vaccine development or Vaccinomics is another powerful innovation which provides a foundation for searching critical determinants of immunity and can promote antigen discovery and the design of novel vaccines for complex pathogens such as the schistosomes. A recent vaccinomics approach for discovering novel schistosome antigens that may not be revealed by conventional proteomics involved the design and manufacture of an immunomics protein microarray, the first to be generated for a multi-cellular pathogen. This vaccine could be administered to children between the ages of 3 and 12 years to prevent severe infection in a particularly high risk population. This review summarizes the current status of Schistosomiasis vaccine development.

2. PREVALENCE OF SCHISTOSOMIASIS AMONG SCHOOL AGE CHILDREN

Uchendu *et al.* (2017) conducted a study aimed towards describing the burden of Schistosomiasis and demographic characteristics among children of migrant workers residing in a rehabilitation home in Ibadan, Nigeria. A cross-sectional study was done using sixty six children and an interviewer-administered questionnaire was used to collect information on demographic and environmental characteristics of the children. The study revealed that the mean age of respondents was 11.8 ± 4.0 years and 57.6% were males. The prevalence of Schistosomiasis was 19.7% with preponderance among males (64.3%) and children aged 12 years and above (71.4%); 85.7% of infected children were from Kwara State; 78.6% waded in water body and 92.9% had red blood cells and pus cells on urine microscopy. The study concluded that the burden of Schistosomiasis was high among school age children of migrant workers and they serve as reservoirs for disease transmission. Also, in a study conducted by Birma *et al.* (2017), Kiri was selected for a comprehensive investigation. The objectives of the study were to determine the prevalence of urinary Schistosomiasis in different communities and the intensity of infection in terms of egg count/10 ml of urine, prevalence among gender and age groups and to relate infection with parent's occupation. A study on the prevalence of urinary Schistosomiasis was conducted in four villages around Kiri Lake in Shelleng Local Government Area, Adamawa State, Nigeria. Two hundred and thirty two urine samples were collected from four randomly selected primary schools from within the four study communities. Overall, prevalence of urinary Schistosomiasis was 48% (111/232), with males recording 49% (69/142) and females 47% (42/90). The total mean egg count (MEC) was 8.3. There was no significant difference in prevalence between males and females ($P > 0.05$). Prevalence was higher among age groups, with the 13–15 year old age group having the highest 62.96% (17/27) and the 4–6 year old age group had the lowest 37% (19/52). There was no statistically significant difference in prevalence among different age groups ($P > 0.05$). Infection was also high among children of fishermen 59.09% (13/22), followed by farmers' children 56.25% (45/80) and the least prevalence was among children of teachers 20% (3/15). Old Banjiram had the highest level of infection 91% (21/23), while Kwadadai had the lowest 36.8% (21/57) ($P < 0.05$). Old Banjiram and children in the 10–12 years age group had the highest MEC of 10.6 and 9.4 respectively. The study revealed a high prevalence of urinary Schistosomiasis among school age children.

3. *SCHISTOSOMA MANSONI* AND *S. HAEMATOBIUM* VACCINE CANDIDATES

Over 100 schistosome vaccine antigens have been identified, of which about a quarter have shown some level of protection in the murine models (Siddiqui *et al.,* 2011). Disappointingly, however, only three molecules, the *S. mansoni* fatty acid binding protein (Sm14), the *S. Mansoni* tetraspanin (Sm-TSP-2) and the *S. haematobium* glutathione S-transferase (Sh28GST), have entered human clinical trials with Smp80 (calpain) undergoing testing in non-human primates (Merrifield *et al.,* 2016). A recent report has suggested that the murine model of Schistosomiasis may be intrinsically flawed for pre-clinical testing of vaccine candidates as a result of the fragility of the pulmonary capillaries in mice which can prevent maturation of a large proportion of schistosome schistosomula upon challenge; which may lead to an incorrect assumption that vaccine antigen-induced acquired protective immunity has been generated (Wilson *et al.,* 2016).

3.1 *S. mansoni* (Sm14)

Schistosomes lack an oxygen-dependent pathway for the synthesis of sterols and fatty acids. Therefore, they are entirely dependent on the mammalian host to provide these essential lipids. Schistosomes use fatty acid binding proteins to absorb, transport and compartmentalize fatty acids from the host and, because of this critical biological function the Sm14 has long been considered a potential vaccine candidate (Tendler *et al.,* 2008). Recombinant Sm14 (rSm14) provided up to 67% protection in terms of reduced *S. mansoni* worm burden in out bred Swiss mice without the use of an adjuvant, and encouragingly, no autoimmune response was observed even though its structure is identical in basic form with the mammalian host homologues (Tendler *et al.,* 1996). It has been shown to be cross-species protective against both *S. mansoni* and *Fasciola hepatica* infection. Development of a dual vaccine effective against both fluke infections has great appeal in terms of human and animal health. The rSm14 with glucopyranosyl lipid adjuvant stable emulsion (GLA-SE) entered and successfully completed a Phase-1 clinical trial in healthy adult volunteers in Brazil, confirming its status as safe and immunogenic vaccine candidate (Santini-Oliveira *et al.,* 2016).

3.2 *Schistosome* 28 kDa *Glutathione S-Transferase*

Schistosome 28 kDa glutathione S-transferase enzymes (28GST) plays a role both in fatty acid metabolism and prostaglandin D2 synthesis and may help the parasite to evade the host immune system (Tebeje *et al.*, 2016). The enzyme present in *S. mansoni* (Sm28GST) has been tested extensively as a recombinant protein vaccine in various experimental models and has shown partial protection in terms of reduction of worm burden, inhibition of female worm fecundity and reduction of egg viability (Capron *et al.*, 2001). Along with Sm14, Sm28GST was one of the six *S. mansoni* antigens originally independently tested under the auspices of TDR/WHO (Bergquist *et al.*, 1998). The *S. haematobium* homologue, Sh28GST (Bilhvax), formulated with alum adjuvant, has undergone human clinical trials (Santini-Oliveira *et al.*, 2016, Bourke *et al.*, 2014). Cytokine production triggered by this vaccine candidate was shown to be influenced by factors such as host age, schistosome infection status and PZQ treatment history, therefore these features should be considered for determining efficacy of the GST-based vaccine during its testing in endemic communities (Bourke *et al.*, 2014). The Phase-1 and 2 clinical trials showed Bilhvax to be safe for both healthy and infected adults and children (Mo *et al.*, 2014). It was scheduled to complete a Phase-3 self-contained, randomized, double blind clinical trial in 2012 evaluating whether co-administration of the vaccine with PZQ could delay pathology due to *S. haematobium* infection in children. The trial results, however, have yet to be released which has raised doubts about the vaccine efficacy (Tebeje *et al.*, 2016).

3.3 *S. mansoni* Calpain (Sm-p80)

Calpain is calcium activated neutral cysteine protease (McManus *et al.*, 2008). Prime-boost vaccination (priming with DNA and boosting with recombinant protein) with Sm-p80, the large subunit of *S. mansoni* calpain, in combination with resiquimod adjuvant, resulted in 49% worm burden reduction, while 50% protection was achieved using the recombinant protein as primary and boost vaccine in mice (Ahmad *et al.*, 2010). With the same approach, but using a different adjuvant, oligo deoxy nucleotide (ODN), 70% worm burden reduction and 75% egg reduction was achieved with the Sm-p80 (Ahmad *et al.*, 2009). Moreover, a 58% worm burden reduction in baboons (*Papio anubis*) was reported recently with the Sm-p80-based vaccine adjuvanted with resiquimod and CpG ODN (Ahmad *et al.*, 2011). Using a different approach, a Sm-p80

DNA vaccine conferred 59% worm burden reduction and 84% decrease in egg production in mice (Ahmad *et al.*, 2009). In baboons the vaccine provided levels of protection against *S. mansoni* infection comparable to those achieved by the irradiated cercarial vaccine; moreover, antibodies and IFN-γ were shown to play an important role in the protective immunity generated in this non-human primate model (Zhang *et al.*, 2010, Ahmad *et al.*, 2009). Importantly, the recombinant Sm-p80 has also been shown to exhibit cross-species protection against *S. haematobium* in both hamsters and baboons (Karmakar *et al.*, 2014). Promisingly, enduring antibody titres were detected in mice at sixty weeks post-vaccination with recombinant Sm-p80, and Sm-p80-specific-IgG for was detected in baboons 5–8 years after initial vaccination with the Sm-80 DNA vaccine (Zhang *et al.*, 2014). It is anticipated that the recombinant Sm-p80/GLA-SE vaccine, "SchistoShield", will move forward to Phase-1 and 2 human clinical trials in 2017 (Karmakar *et al.*, 2014, Zhang *et al.*, 2014). Furthermore, it has also been shown that Sm-p80 has a therapeutic effect in vaccinated baboons through decreasing the numbers of established worms, reducing the retention of eggs in tissues, and decreasing the number of eggs excreted in faeces (Karmakar *et al.*, 2014).

3.4 *S. mansoni* Tetraspanins (Sm-TSP-2)

The tetraspanins are a group of proteins that are highly abundant in the schistosome tegument where they are found at the outer-most membrane of the intra-mammalian stage of the parasite, hence are highly exposed to the host immune system (Braschi *et al.*, 2006). The major *S. mansoni* tetraspanin are Sm-TSP-1 and Sm-TSP-2 with the latter conferring protection in *S. mansoni* challenge animal models and also correlating with protective immunity in naturally resistant people (Loukas *et al.*, 2007).

3.5 *S. mansoni* 29 (Sm29)

Sm29 is present in the tegument of adult worms and schistosomula and in its recombinant form it induces high level production of both the IgG1 and IgG3 isotypes among individuals resistant to infection and re-infection (Cardoso *et al.*, 2006). There are reports that recombinant Sm29 can prevent infection in animals previously exposed to *S. mansoni*. For example, 26–48% protection was observed in BALB/c mice that were previously infected with a Brazilian strain of *S. mansoni* and treated with PZQ (Alves *et al.*, 2015). Recently an increased level of protection was obtained through combining Sm29 with Sm14 in the presence of poly

I:C adjuvant; 40.3, 68.2 and 57.9% reductions in adult worm burden, liver egg burden and intestinal eggs, respectively, whereas achieved, along with a reduction in granuloma size and number in livers of immunized mice (Ewaisha *et al.*, 2014). Another report showed that by fusing Sm29 and Sm14, a 48.4% reduction in worm burden was achieved in mice (Mossallam *et al.*, 2015). In a further advance, when the recombinant Sm29 was subjected to high hydrostatic pressure which dissociated the aggregated protein resulting in a successfully folded, soluble, stable and structured molecule, it was protective against *S. mansoni*, thereby paving the way for its industrial production down track (Chura-Chambi *et al.*, 2013).

4. ANTIOXIDANTS

The antioxidants Cu–Zn superoxide dismutase (SOD) and glutathione S peroxidase (GPX) induced ≥ 40% reduction in worm burdens when administered as DNA-based vaccines in *S. mansoni*-challenged mice (Shalaby *et al.*, 2003). Similarly, a recent study showed a protective effect against Schistosomiasis in baboons (Carvalho-Queiroz *et al.*, 2015). Vaccinated baboons with two different formulations of SOD (SmCT-SOD and SmSP-SOD) and one of GPX, with a protocol of priming with naked DNA and boosting with the respective recombinant antioxidant proteins encapsulated in polylactic acid microspheres, exhibited a robust immune response, which resulted in a reduction in worm numbers, and pronounced anti-pathology effect compared with control animals.

5. DIGESTIVE TRACT PROTEINS

S. mansoni worms ingest host blood which passes through the oesophagus before arriving at an area in the gut where many peptidases catalyse its proteolysis. Processing of the blood and the resulting uptake of nutrients are functions essential for the survival of the parasite (Tebeje *et al.*, 2016). Blocking these critical processes represents an important strategy for vaccine development and a number of digestive tract proteins, that are not recognized by host immune responses during normal infection, but are essential for parasite survival, have been tested as cryptic vaccine candidates (Figueiredo *et al.*, 2015). One example was the trialling of a soluble form of schistosome lysosome-associated membrane glycoprotein, located in the gastrodermis, which resulted in reduction in worm burden (16–25%) and in faecal eggs (52–60%); moreover, its insoluble form produced up to 38% reduction in liver egg burden (Nawaratna *et al.*, 2015). Another recent study identified a number of esophageal secreted proteins, encoded by micro exon genes (MEGs), that are involved in the initial processing of ingested blood and these, along with lysosomal hydrolase, also localised to the oesophagus, may prove to be novel immune targets (Wilson *et al.*, 2015).

5.1 *S. japonicum* (Sj97)

Paramyosin is a myofibrillar 97 kDa protein present in the muscle layers and the tegument of schistosomes that has long been regarded as a vaccine candidate against both *S. japonicum* and *S. mansoni* infection (McManus *et al.*, 2008). An early study showed that mice vaccinated intra peritoneal with purified paramyosin (without use of an adjuvant) stimulated 62–86% resistances against *S. japonicum* cercarial challenge (Ramirez *et al.*, 1996). In addition to preventing infection, a longitudinal treatment-re-infection design study in Leyte, the Philippines showed that a Th2 bias in response to Sj97 predicted a longer time to human re-infection and lower re-infection intensity after treatment with PZQ (Leenstra *et al.*, 2006, Jiz *et al.*, 2015). Moreover, it was reported in the human Leyte cohort that individuals who produce IgE but not IgG4 in response to rSj97 had 77% lower re-infection intensity after 12 months of treatment with PZQ (Jiz *et al.*, 2009 and 2015).

5.2 *S. japonicum* 26 kDa GST *plasmid* DNA Vaccine (Sj26GST)

A *S. japonicum* 26 kDa GST plasmid DNA vaccine (Sj26GST) resulted in a significant reduction in worm numbers, hepatic and faecal eggs in vaccinated mice (Wei *et al.*, 2008). When the DNA vaccine was given in combination with interleukin 18 (IL-18), a potent IFN-γ inducing factor, the protective efficacy was improved. DNA vaccines have some advantages over other types of immunization but they have some limitations concerning the gene delivery system. A recent study reported on a novel nanoparticle formulation of the Sj26GST DNA vaccine; although there was no significant reduction in worm burden, a highly significant decline in tissue egg burden and fecundity of female worms were recorded (Mbanefo *et al.*, 2015). Toll-like receptor (TLR) 7/8 ligands (*e.g.* R848) and TLR 9 ligands (*e.g.* CpG oligodeoxynucleotides, or CpG) as adjuvants can increase vaccine effectiveness through activating the innate immune system and ultimately activating and directing the adaptive immune system. Such adjuvants have been shown to potentiate the activity of the Sj26GST DNA vaccine in mice by increasing splenocyte proliferation, elevating IgG,

IgG2a, IFNγ and TNFα levels, and preventing Treg-mediated immune-suppression (Wang *et al.,* 2013). In another development, Sj26GST alone, or in combination with the *S. japonicum* fatty acid binding protein, expressed in recombinant pseudorabies virus (PRV) Bartha-K61, induced significant levels of specific immunity and protection in mice and, importantly, sheep, emphasising the potential effectiveness of this live vector for vaccination against *S. japonica* in animal reservoirs (Wei *et al.,* 2010).

5.3 *S. japonicum* Triose-Phosphate Isomerase

The glycolytic pathway enzyme triose-phosphate isomerase (TPI) is expressed in all stages of the schistosome life-cycle and represents another targeted vaccine candidate for *S. japonica.* An early study showed that a *S. japonicum* (Chinese strain) TPI (SjCTPI) plasmid DNA vaccine (with or without an IL-12 DNA plasmid) protected pigs against challenge infection. Synergistic enhancement of immunogenicity and protection in mice against *S. japonicum* challenge was achieved with codon optimization and electroporation delivery of the SjTPI DNA (Zhu *et al.,* 2006), showing a similar level of protection as a replication-defective recombinant optimized SjTPI adenoviral vaccine (Dai *et al.,* 2014) which was enhanced using a heterologous prime-boost strategy (Dai *et al.,* 2015). A study, conducted in Chinese water buffalo with a DNA vaccine encoding SjCTPI alone or fused with bovine HSP-70 with booster immunizations co-administered using a plasmid encoding IL-12, resulted in a significant reduction in worm numbers, liver and faecal eggs and in faecal miracidial hatching (Da'dara *et al.,* 2008). SjCTPI, delivered by a heterologous "prime-boost" regimen, has been used to vaccinate bovines in China as part of a multi-component integrated control package (Gray *et al.,* 2014).

5.4 *S. japonicum* Insulin Receptors

S. japonicum possess two types of insulin receptors (SjIRs) which, on binding to mammalian host insulin, can activate the parasite's insulin pathway, which is pivotal for glucose uptake, growth, and maturation (You *et al.,* 2010). Recombinant ligands of both *S. japonicum* insulin receptor 1 and 2 (SjLD1, SjLD2), tested in vaccine/challenge trials in mice resulted in significant reductions in faecal eggs output, mature intestinal eggs and stunting of adult worms (You *et al.,* 2012, You *et al.,* 2015). The retardation in growth of the worms likely resulted from reduced glucose uptake (You *et al.,* 2012). Furthermore, knockdown of the SjIRs using

RNA interference (RNAi) resulted in their reduced expression coupled with a reduction in the transcription level of downstream genes within the insulin pathway that are associated with glucose metabolism and schistosome fecundity (You *et al.*, 2015), thereby reinforcing their vaccine potential.

5.5 *S. japonicum* (Sj14)

In early studies, Sj14 (fatty acid binding protein; SjFABP), the *S. japonicum* homologue of Sm14, generated no or only a limited level of protection (McManus *et al.*, 2008), but when given to mice as a DNA vaccine with a plasmid coding for IL-18 as adjuvant, the level of protection was increased substantially (Wei *et al.*, 2009). The latter study also showed that SjFABP + IL-18 increased the Th1 immune response by inducing a higher level of IFNγ and a lower level of IL-4 compared with mice vaccinated only with SjFABP alone (Wei *et al.*, 2009). Somewhat disappointingly, the Sj14 DNA vaccine, coupled with the Sj26GST a bivalent DNA vaccine, resulted in reduction in the level of protective compared to that obtained by the monovalent DNA immunization (Tu *et al.*, 2014).

5.6 *S. japonicum* (Sj23)

Sj23, like Sm-TSP-2, a member of the tetraspanin family, is a 23-kDa surface-exposed integral membrane protein expressed in all parasite stages. It was shown in BALB/c mice to elicit a rapid humoral immune response dominated by IgG2a antibodies, but not IgG1, and did not provide protection against cercarial challenge after priming with recombinant Semliki forest virus particles followed by a boost with the recombinant Sj23 (Jiang *et al.*, 2010). A subsequent report of mice vaccinated with purified recombinant protein LHD Sj23-GST (large hydrophilic domain of Sj23 fused with Sj26GST) in combination with one of three adjuvants (Freund's adjuvant, FA), Montanide ISA 206 or Montanide ISA 70 M), and parasite challenged, resulted in high-level production of LHDSj23-GST-specific IgG1, IgG2a and IgG3 antibodies and significant reductions in worm burden (Zhu *et al.*, 2012). In order to further improve the level of protection, a multivalent DNA vaccine comprising Sj23, glyceraldedyde-3 phosphate dehydrogenase (SjGAPDH), SjFABP and Sj26 was tested in mice which resulted in very high levels of protective efficacy in terms of reduction in worm burden (70.8%) and liver eggs (60.7%) (Zhu *et al.*, 2011). Another study in mice, using three cocktail DNA vaccines encoding Sj23, SjCTPI and NP30, boosted by electroporation *in-vivo* and a protein vaccine boost to this regimen, resulted in 60% reduction in worm numbers and more than 60% reduction in the liver egg burden (Dai *et al.,* 2009).

6. NEW ANTIGEN DISCOVERY: A WAY FORWARD

New antigen discovery has been aided by major recent advances in schistosome genomics, transcriptomics and post-genomic technologies (Ricciardi *et al.,* 2015). Proteomics is another important and now widely used tool that can identify potential vaccine targets with focus on protein constituents of different schistosome sources such as host-parasite interface comprising tegument or gut. Studies on the tegument have used a number of procedures including biotin-labelling of live parasites and subsequent isolation and characterisation of the biotinylated proteins using tandem mass spectrometry (MS/MS) to identify surface-located proteins, and therefore those accessible to host antibodies. Proteomics of the schistosomegut and its contents has shed new light on the functionality of this important region of the parasite (Driguez *et al.,* 2016).

Coupled with other approaches such as metabolomics, interrogation of the schistosome proteome, particularly the surface, provides a mechanism to identify important clinically-relevant proteins and those having potential as new vaccine targets (De Sousa *et al.*, 2016). A recent vaccinomics approach for discovering novel schistosome antigens that may not be revealed by conventional proteomics involved the design and manufacture of an immunomics protein microarray, the first to be generated for a multi-cellular pathogen. Mostly surface-derived proteins (215 in total) from *S. japonicum* and *S. mansoni* were selected and they were produced using a rapid *in-vitro* translation system, and then printed as a vaccine discovery tool (Driguez *et al.,* 2010 and 2016, Mc William *et al.,* 2012). The reactivity of microarray proteins can be measured with anti-sera from human patients or Schistosomiasis-resistant/exposed animals using a labelled secondary antibody and a laser microarray scanner; highly reactive proteins are then assessed as putative vaccines. One application of the array used antibodies from acutely- or chronically-infected Chinese individuals with early/advanced *S. japonicum*, and subjects exposed, but stool negative for *S. japonicum* eggs, for screening. This resulted in identification of 25 immuno dominant antigens, including a number of vaccine candidates, transporters, tetraspanin-related proteins, and unannotated proteins (Driguez *et al.,* 2016). The array has also been screened for IgG subclassess and IgE responses, using sera from a human Brazilian cohort of putatively resistant (PR) and chronically *S. mansoni*-infected (CI) individuals stratified by worm intensity levels (high, medium, low), determined by faecal egg counts, so as to identify antibody signatures reflective of protective *vs* non-protective immune responses (Gaze *et al.,* 2014). Probing for IgE responses allowed identification of antigens that might induce potentially deleterious hypersensitivity reactions if used as subunit vaccines in endemic populations so it was encouraging that the PR individuals did not mount an intense IgE response to these antigens compared with CI subjects. Using this immunomics-based approach to Schistosomiasis vaccine antigen discovery was further validated by identification of targets of protective IgG1 immune response in PZQ-induced resistant subjects exposed to *S. haematobium*; uncharacterized proteins and a number of recognised vaccine antigens (*e.g.* glucose transporters, tetraspanins, glutathione-S-transferases, calpain) were identified (Pearson *et al.,* 2015). The same report described use of sera from *Rhesus macaques* experimentally rendered resistant to *S. japonicum* infection to screen for antigen targets, and discovery of new and known vaccine candidates, including many recognized by the human subjects. Another important application has been the immune screening of the schistosome microarray with antibody secreting cell (ASC)-probes (Driguez *et al.,* 2010 and 2016, McWilliam *et al.,* 2012), generated from lymph nodes draining the sites of larval *S. Japonicum* migration (McWilliam *et al.,* 2013). This technique is especially advantageous for recognizing antigens with low immunogenicity (selective pressure may have an influence on important protective epitopes which evolve over time with low immunogenicity) or those only temporarily exposed to the immune response (McWilliam *et al.,* 2012). In one study, ASC probes (from skin and lung) and sera from semi-permissive rats and from susceptible mice were used to screen the array after infection and re-infection with *S. japonicum* (Driguez *et al.,* 2016). A total of 29 antigens, including a number of recognised vaccine candidates and several *S. japonicum* homologues of human Schistosomiasis resistance markers—the tegument allergen-like proteins—were differentially recognized by infected hosts from which eight proteins were prioritized as putative novel schistosome vaccine candidates and diagnostic antigens (Driguez *et al.,* 2016). In a related study, the protein microarray, screened with ASC probes generated from *S. Japonicum* infected rats, resulted in the identification of a novel antigen, termed *S. japonicum* Ly-6-like protein 1 (Sj-L6L-1) which shares structural and sequence features with the Ly-6 protein family and has several other features suggesting it is a promising vaccine candidate against developing larvae *S. japonicum* larvae (McWilliam *et al.,* 2014).

7. CONCLUSIONS

Schistosomiasis remains a substantial public health problem due to the very high levels of morbidity it causes in many parts of the world especially in Nigeria. School age children who live in areas with water bodies that harbour the snail intermediate host are most susceptible to the diseases and they serve as reservoirs for transmission of the disease. Currently, the treatment is entirely dependent on PZQ chemotherapy. As exclusive use of one drug may lead to emergence of drug resistant strains, development and deployment of a vaccine as part of an integrated approach for prevention and control of Schistosomiasisis is to be encouraged. Much of our current understanding of immunity and immune mechanisms against Schistosomiasis rely on studies conducted on mice, but vaccines based on studies performed only in mouse model could have undesirable effects if taken prematurely to human clinical trials. The recent concern raised about using mice for determining efficacy of vaccine candidates further reinforces the argument that additional critical examination of any identified candidate vaccine antigen, whether or not it has foundation in acquired immunity is essential, and that moving to studies using larger models such as rabbits, pigs or bovines in the case of *S. japonicum*, or non-human primates for *S. mansoni* and *S. haematobium,* is clearly necessary. Similarly, protection levels of many candidate vaccines show improvement after modification of antigen formulation and upon using improved delivery systems. Combining different genes or antigens can also result in higher levels of vaccine-induced protection with some exception. Targeting key biological functions of schistosomes such as tegumental integrity, fecundity, and nutrient uptake using RNAi represent key potential sites identify vaccine candidates (Gobert *et al.*, 2014). Although in its infancy, CRISPR technology may provide a novel approach identifying specific protein-encoding schistosomegenes for vaccine candidate discovery (Cai *et al.,* 2016). Schistosomiasis vaccine development has proven highly challenging and costly and new funding mechanisms are required to promote generation of anti-schistosome vaccines pipeline, similar to that in place for many other infectious diseases, and to progress the existing promising candidates into clinical trials. It is becoming apparent that mass drug administration alone will not eliminate Schistosomiasis and that a vaccine will likely be a key component of an integrated approach of any future Schistosomiasis control intervention toolbox.

REFERENCES

[1] Ahmad G., Torben W., Zhang W., Wyatt M. and Siddiqui A.A. (2009). Sm-p80-based DNA vaccine formulation induces potent protective immunity against *Schistosoma mansoni. Parasite Immunology* 31: 156–161.

[2] Ahmad G., Zhang W., Torben W., Ahrorov A., Damian R.T. and Wolf R.F. (2011). Preclinical prophylactic efficacy testing of Sm-p80-based vaccine in a nonhuman primate model of *Schistosoma mansoni* infection and immunoglobulin G and E responses to Sm-p80 in human serum samples from an area where Schistosomiasis is endemic. *Journal of Infectious Diseases* 204: 1437–49.

[3] Ahmad G., Zhang W., Torben W., Damian R.T., Wolf RF., White G.L. (2009). Protective and antifecundity effects of Sm-p80-based DNA vaccine formulation against *Schistosoma mansoni* in a nonhuman primate model. *Vaccine* 27: 2830–2837.

[4] Ahmad G., Zhang W., Torben W., Haskins C., Diggs S. and Noor Z. (2009). Prime-boost and recombinant protein vaccination strategies using Sm-p80 protects against *Schistosomamansoni* infection in the mouse model to levels previously attainable only by the irradiated cercarial vaccine. *Parasitology Research* 105: 1767–1777.

[5] Ahmad G., Zhang W., Torben W., Noor Z. and Siddiqui A.A. (2010). Protective effects of Sm-p80 in the presence of resiquimod as an adjuvant against challenge infection with *Schistosoma mansoni* in mice. *International Journal on Infectious Diseases* 14: 781–787.

[6] Alves C.C., Araujo N., dos Santos V.C., Couto F.B., Assis N.R. and Morais S.B. (2015). Sm29, but not Sm22.6 retains its ability to induce a protective immune response in mice previously exposed to a *Schistosoma mansoni* infection. *PLoS Neglected Tropical Diseases* 9:e0003537.

[7] Angaye T.C. (2016). A review on the epidemiology and control of Schistosomiasis in Nigeria. *Journal of Medical Health Research* 1: 1–23.

[8] Beaumier C.M., Gillespie P.M., Hotez P.J., Bottazzi M.E. (2013). New vaccines for neglected parasitic diseases and dengue. *Transl Res* 162: 144–55.

[9] Bergquist N.R. and Colley D.G. (1998). Schistosomiasis vaccine: research to development. *Parasitology Today* 14: 99–104.

[10] Birma J.S., Chessed G., Shadrach P.A., Nganjiwa J.I., Yako A.B., Vandi P., Laurat T. (2017). Urinary Schistosomiasis in communities around Kiri Lake, Shelleng Local Government Area, Adamawa State, Nigeria. *Journal of Applied Science and Environmental Management* 21:128–134.

[11] Bourke C.D., Nausch N., Rujeni N., Appleby L.J., Trottein F. and Midzi N. (2014). Cytokine responses to the anti-schistosome vaccine candidate antigen glutathione-S-transferase vary with host age and are boosted by praziquantel treatment. *PLoS Neglected Tropical Diseases* 8: e2846.

[12] Braschi S., Borges W.C., Wilson R.A. (2006). Proteomic analysis of the schistosome tegument and its surface membranes. Cruz Institute 101: 205–212.

[13] Cai P., Gobert G.N., You H., McManus D.P. (2016). The Tao survivorship of schistosomes: implications for Schistosomiasis control. *Int J Parasitol* 46: 453–463.

[14] Capron A., Capron M., Dombrowicz D. and Riveau G. (2001). Vaccine strategies against Schistosomiasis: from concepts to clinical trials. *Intl Arch Allergy Immunology* 124: 9–15.

[15] Capron A., Riveau U. (2002). Vaccine development against Schistosomiasis from concepts to clinical trials. *British Med Bull* 62: 139–148.

[16] Cardoso F.C., Pacifico R.N., Mortara R.A. and Oliveira S.C. (2006). Human antibody responses of patients living in endemic areas for Schistosomiasis to the tegumental protein Sm29 identified through genomic studies. *Clin Exp Immunol* 144: 382–391.

[17] Carvalho-Queiroz C., Nyakundi R., Ogongo P., Rikoi H., Egilmez N.K., Farah I.O., *et al.* (2015). Protective potential of antioxidant enzymes as vaccines for Schistosomiasis in a non-human primate model. *Front Immunol* 6: 273.

[18] Central Intelligence Agency (2015). Nigeria in the world factbook. https://www.cia.gov/library/publications/the-world-factbook/geos/ni.html

[19] Chura-Chambi R.M., Nakajima E., de Carvalho R.R., Miyasato P.A., Oliveira S.C., Morganti L. (2013). Refolding of the recombinant protein Sm29, a step toward the production of the vaccine candidate against Schistosomiasis. *Journal of Biotechnology* 168: 511–519.

[20] Cioli D., Pica-Mattoccia L., Basso A. and Guidi A. (2014). Schistosomiasis control: praziquantel forever? *Molecular Biochemistry and Parasitology* 195: 23–29.

[21] Curti E., Kwityn C., Zhan B., Gillespie P., Brelsford J. and Deumic V. (2013). Expression at a 20 L scale and purification of the extracellular domain of the *Schistosoma mansoni* TSP-2 recombinant protein: a vaccine candidate for human intestinal Schistosomiasis. *Hum Vaccin Immunother* 9: 2342–2350.

[22] Da'dara A.A., Li Y.S., Xiong T., Zhou J., Williams G.M., McManus D.P., *et al.* (2008). DNA-based vaccines protect against zoonotic Schistosomiasis in water buffalo. *Vaccine* 26: 3617–3625.

[23] Dai Y., Wang X., Tang J., Zhao S., Xing Y., Dai J., *et al.* (2015). Enhancement of protective efficacy through adenoviral vectored vaccine priming and protein boosting strategy encoding triosephosphate isomerase (SjTPI) against *Schistosoma japonicum* in mice. *PLoS One* 10: e0120792.

[24] Dai Y., Wang X., Zhao S., Tang J., Zhang L., Dai J., *et al.* (2014). Construction and evaluation of replication-defective recombinant optimized triosephosphate isomerase adenoviral vaccination in *Schistosoma japonicum* challenged mice. Vaccine 32: 771–778.

[25] Dai Y., Zhu Y., Harn D.A., Wang X., Tang J., Zhao S., *et al.* (2009). DNA vaccination by electroporation and boosting with recombinant proteins enhances the efficacy of DNA vaccines for *Schistosomiasis japonica. Clin Vaccine Immunol* 16:1796–1803.

[26] De Sousa K.P., Doolan D.L. (2016). Immunomics: a 21st century approach to vaccine development for complex pathogens. *Parasitology* 143: 236–244.

[27] Diemert D.J., Pinto A.G., Freire J., Jariwala A., Santiago H. and Hamilton R.G. (2012). Generalized urticaria induced by the Na-ASP-2 hookworm

vaccine: implications for the development of vaccines against helminths. *Journal of Allergy Clinical Immunology* 130:169–176.

[28] Driguez P., Doolan D.L., Loukas A., Felgner P.L., McManus D.P. (2010). Schistosomiasis vaccine discovery using immunomics. *Parasit Vectors* 3: 4.

[29] Driguez P., Li Y., Gaze S., Pearson M.S., Nakajima R., Trieu A., *et al.* (2016). Antibody signatures reflect different disease pathologies in patients with Schistosomiasis due to *Schistosoma japonicum*. *Journal of Infectious Diseases* 213:122–130.

[30] Driguez P., McManus D.P., Gobert G.N. (2016). Clinical implications of recent findings in schistosome proteomics. *Expert Rev Proteomics* 13:19–33.

[31] Driguez P., McWilliam H.E., Gaze S., Piedrafita D., Pearson M.S., Nakajima R., *et al.* (2016). Specific humoral response of hosts with variable Schistosomiasis susceptibility. *Immunol Cell Biol* 94: 52–65.

[32] Enersen O.D. (2010). Theodore Maximillian Bilharz. http://www.whonameedit.com/doctor.cfm/2829.html. Accessed 23rd April, 2015.

[33] Ewaisha R.E., Bahey-El-Din M., Mossallam S.F., Amer E.I., Aboushleib H.M. and Khalil A.M. (2014). Combination of the two schistosomal antigens Sm14 and Sm29 elicits significant protection against experimental *Schistosoma mansoni* infection. *Experimental Parasitology* 145: 51–60.

[34] Federal Ministry of Health (2015). Report on epidemiological mapping of Schistosomiasis and soil transmitted Helminthiasis in 19 states and the FCT, Nigeria. www.health.gov.ng/doc/SchistoSTH.pdf.

[35] Figueiredo B.C., Ricci N.D., de Assis N.R., de Morais S.B., Fonseca C.T., Oliveira S.C. (2015). Kicking in the guts: *Schistosoma mansoni* digestive tract proteins are potential candidates for vaccine development. *Front Immunol* 6: 22.

[36] Gaze S., Driguez P., Pearson M.S., Mendes T., Doolan D.L., Trieu A., *et al.* (2014). An immunomics approach to schistosome antigen discovery: antibody signatures of naturally resistant and chronically infected individuals from endemic areas. *PLoS Pathog* 10: e1004033.

[37] Gobert G.N., You H., McManus D.P. (2014). Gaining biological perspectives from schistosome genomes. Mol *Biochem Parasitol* 196: 21–28.

[38] Goncalves De Assis N.R., Batistoni de Morais S., Figueiredo B.C., Ricci N.D., de Almeida L.A., da Silva Pinheiro C. (2015). DNA Vaccine encoding the chimeric form of *Schistosoma mansoni* Sm-TSP2 and Sm29 confers partial protection against challenge infection. *PLoS One* 10: e0125075.

[39] Gray D.J., Li Y.S., Williams G.M., Zhao Z.Y., Harn D.A., Li S.M., *et al.* (2014). A multi-component integrated approach for the elimination of Schistosomiasis in the People's Republic of China: design and baseline results of a 4-year cluster-randomised intervention trial. *Int J Parasitol* 44:659–668.

[40] Hotez P., Molyneux D., Fenwick A., Kumaresan J., Sachs S., Sachs J., *et al.* (2007). Control of neglected tropical diseases. *N + J Med* 357:1018–1027.

[41] Jiang N., Cai P., Yin J., Hao L., Lu H., Wang X., *et al.* (2010). Characterization of antibody responses to the Sj23 antigen of *Schistosoma japonicum* after infection and immunization. *Acta Trop* 116: 9–14.

[42] Jiz M., Friedman J.F., Leenstra T., Jarilla B., Pablo A., Langdon G., *et al.* (2009). Immunoglobulin E (IgE) responses to paramyosin predict resistance to reinfection with *Schistosoma japonicum* and are attenuated by IgG4. *Infect Immun* 77: 2051–2058.

[43] Jiz M.A., Wu H., Olveda R., Jarilla B., Kurtis J.D. (2015). Development of paramyosin as a vaccine candidate for Schistosomiasis. *Front Immunol* 6: 347.

[44] Karmakar S., Zhang W., Ahmad G., Torben W., Alam M.U., Le L., *et al.*, Cross-species protection: *Schistosoma mansoni* Sm-p80 vaccine confers protecttion against *Schistosoma haematobium* in hamsters and baboons. Vaccine 32: 1296–1303.

[45] Karmakar S., Zhang W., Ahmad G., Torben W., Alam M.U. and Le L. (2014). Use of a Sm-p80-based therapeutic vaccine to kill established adult schistosome parasites in chronically infected baboons. *Journal of Infectious Diseases*; 209(12):1929–40.

[46] Leenstra T, Acosta LP, Wu HW, Langdon GC, Solomon JS, Manalo DL, *et al.*, T-helper-2 cytokine responses to Sj97 predict resistance to reinfection with *Schistosoma japonicum*. Infect Immun. 2006; 74(1):370–81.

[47] Loukas A., Tran M. and Pearson M.S. (2007). Schistosome membrane proteins as vaccines. *International Journal of Parasitology* 37: 257–263.

[48] Mbanefo E.C., Kumagai T., Kodama Y., Kurosaki T., Furushima-Shimogawara R., Cherif M.S. *et al.* (2015). Immunogenicity and anti-fecundity effect of nanoparticle coated glutathione S-transferase (SjGST) DNA vaccine against murine *Schistosoma japonicum* infection. *Parasitol Intl* 64: 24–31.

[49] McManus D.P. and Loukas A. (2008). Current status of vaccines for Schistosomiasis. *Clinical Microbiology Revised* 21: 225–242.

[50] McWilliam H.E., Driguez P., Piedrafita D., Maupin K.A., Haab B.B., McManus D.P., *et al.* (2013). The developing schistosome worms elicit distinct immune responses in different tissue regions. *Immunol Cell Biol* 91: 477–485.

[51] McWilliam H.E., Driguez P., Piedrafita D., McManus D.P., Meeusen E.N. (2014). Discovery of novel *Schistosoma japonicum* antigens using a targeted protein microarray approach. *Parasite Vectors* 7: 290.

[52] McWilliam H.E., Driguez P., Piedrafita D., McManus D.P., Meeusen E.N. (2012). Novel immunomic technologies for schistosome vaccine development. *Parasite Immunol* 34: 276–284.

[53] Merrifield M., Hotez P.J., Beaumier C.M., Gillespie P., Strych U., Hayward T. (2016). Advancing a vaccine to prevent human Schistosomiasis. *Vaccine* 34: 2988–2991.

[54] Mo A.X., Agosti J.M., Walson J.L., Hall B.F. and Gordon L. (2014). Schistosomiasis elimination strategies and potential role of a vaccine in achieving global health goals. *America Journal of Tropical Medical Hygiene* 90:54–60.

[55] Mossallam S.F., Amer E.I., Ewaisha R.E., Khalil A.M., Aboushleib H.M. and Bahey-El-Din M. (2015). Fusion protein comprised of the two schistosomal antigens, Sm14 and Sm29, provides significant protection against *Schistosoma mansoni* in murine infection model. *BMC Infectious Diseases* 15: 147.

[56] Nawaratna S.S., Gobert G.N., Willis C., Mulvenna J., Hofmann A., McManus D.P., *et al.* (2015). Lysosome-associated membrane glycoprotein (LAMP) – preliminary study on a hidden antigen target for vaccination against Schistosomiasis. *Sci Rep* 5: 15069.

[57] Nwosu D.C., Nwachukwu P.C., Avoaja D.A., Ajero C.M.U., Nwanjo H.U., Obeagu E.I., Nnorom R.M., Okpara K.E. and Kanu S.N. (2015). Index of potential contamination for urinary Schistosomiasis in Afikpo North L.G.A. Ebonyi State, Nigeria. *Europe Journal of Biomedicine and Pharmacology Science* 2: 439–450.

[58] Oketch-Rabah H.A. and Dossaji S.F. (1998). Molluscicides of plant origin: Molluscicidal activity of some Kenyan medicinal plants. *South African Journal of Science* 94: 299–301.

[59] Okoli E.I., Odaibo A.B. (1999). Urinary Schistosomiasis among school children in Ibadan, an urban community in southern Nigeria. *Trop Med Intl Hlth* 4: 308–315.

[60] Okpala H.O. (2010). Epidemiological studies of Schistosomiasis in Jos South Local Government Area, Plateau state, Nigeria. University of Jos, http://irepos.unijos.edu.ng/jspui/bitstream/123456789/190/1/Epidemiological%20Studies.pdf.

[61] Pearson, M.S., Becker, L., Driguez, P., Young, N. D., Gaze, S., Mendes, T. Of monkeys and men: immunomic profiling of sera from humans and non-human primates resistant to Schistosomiasis reveals novel potential vaccine candidates. Front Immunol. 2015; 6:213.

[62] Pinheiro C.S., Ribeiro A.P., Cardoso F.C., Martins V.P., Figueiredo B.C. and Assis N.R. (2014). A multivalent chimeric vaccine composed of *Schistosoma mansoni* SmTSP-2 and Sm29 was able to induce protection against infection in mice. *Parasite Immunology* 36: 303–312.

[63] Ramirez B.L., Kurtis J.D., Wiest P.M., Arias P., Aligui F., Acosta L., *et al.* (1996). Paramyosin: a candidate vaccine antigen against *Schistosoma japonicum. Parasite Immunology* 18: 49–52.

[64] Ricciardi A., Ndao M. (2015). Still hope for Schistosomiasis vaccine. *Hum Vaccin Immunother* 11: 2504–2508.

[65] Ross A.G., Olveda R.M., Acosta L., Harn D.A., Chy D. and Li Y. (2013). Road to the elimination of Schistosomiasis from Asia: the journey is far from over. *Microbes Infections* 15: 858–865.

[66] Santini-Oliveira M., Coler R.N., Parra J., Veloso V., Jayashankar L. and Pinto P.M. (2016). Schistosomiasis vaccine candidate Sm14/GLA-SE: Phase 1 safety and immunogenicity clinical trial in healthy, male adults. *Vaccine* 34: 586–594.

[67] Shalaby K.A., Yin L., Thakur A., Christen L., Niles E.G., LoVerde P.T. (2003). Protection against *Schistosoma mansoni* utilizing DNA vaccination with genes encoding Cu/Zn cytosolic superoxide dismutase, signal peptide-containing superoxide dismutase and glutathione peroxidase enzymes. *Vaccine* 22: 130–136.

[68] Siddiqui A.A., Siddiqui B.A., Ganley-Leal L. (2011). Schistosomiasis vaccines. *Human Vaccines* 7:1192–1197.

[69] Stanford University (2015). The history of Schistosomiasis in Nigeria. 2015. schisto.stanford.edu/pdf/Nigeria.pdf.

[70] Stephenson R., You H., McManus D.P., Toth I. (2014). Schistosome vaccine adjuvants in preclinical and clinical research. Vaccines 2: 654–685.

[71] Sturrock R.F. (2001). Schistosomiasis epidemiology and control: how did we get here and where should we go? Cruz Institute 96(Suppl): 17–27.

[72] Sulivan J.T., Cheng T.C. and Rowland K.H. (1984). Milotic responses of the anterior pericardial wail of *Biomphalaria glabrata* (Mollusca) subjected to challenge. *Journal of Invertebrate Pathology* 44: 114–116.

[73] Tebeje B.M., Harvie M., You H., Loukas A., McManus D.P. (2016). Schistosomiasis vaccines: where do we stand? *Parasites & Vectors* 9: 528.

[74] Tendler M. Simpson A.J. (2008). The biotechnology-value chain: development of Sm14 as a Schistosomiasis vaccine. *Acta Tropica* 108: 263–266.

[75] Tendler M., Brito C.A., Vilar M.M., Serra-Freire N., Diogo C.M. Almeida M.S. (1996). A *Schistosoma mansoni* fatty acid-binding protein, Sm14, is the potential basis of a dual-purpose anti-helminth vaccine. *Proc Natl Acad Sci* 93: 269–273.

[76] Tendler M., Almeida M. Simpson A. (2015). Development of the Brazilian anti Schistosomiasis vaccine based on the recombinant fatty acid binding protein Sm14 plus GLA-SE adjuvant. *Front Immunology* 6: 218.

[77] Tu Y., Hu Y., Fan G., Chen Z., Liu L., Man D., *et al.* (2014). Protective effects of membrane-anchored and secreted DNA vaccines encoding fatty acid-binding protein and glutathione S-transferase against *Schistosoma japonicum*. *PLoS One* 9: e86575.

[78] Uchendu O., Oladoyin V., Idowu M., Adeyera O., Olabisi O., Oluwatosin O. Leigh G. (2017). Urinary Schistosomiasis among vulnerable children in a rehabilitation home in Ibadan, Oyo state, Nigeria. *BMC Infectious Diseases* 17: 2591–2596.

[79] Uneke C., Ugwuok-Adibuah S., Nwakpu K., Ngwu B. (2010). An assessment of *Schistosoma haematobium* infection and urinary tract bacterial infection amongst school children in rural eastern Nigeria. *Intl J Lab Med* 4: 1.

[80] Wang X., Dong L., Ni H., Zhou S., Xu Z., Hoellwarth J.S., *et al.* (2013). Combined TLR7/8 and TLR9 ligands potentiate the activity of a *Schistosoma japonicum* DNA vaccine. *PLoS Negl Trop Dis* 7: e2164.

[81] Wei F., Liu Q., Gao S., Shang L., Zhai Y., Men J., *et al.* (2008). Enhancement by IL-18 of the protective effect of a *Schistosoma japonicum* 26 kDa GST plasmid DNA vaccine in mice. *Vaccine* 26: 4145–4149.

[82] Wei F., Liu Q., Zhai Y., Fu Z., Liu W., Shang L., *et al.* (2009). IL-18 enhances protective effect in mice immunized with a Schistosoma japonicum FABP DNA vaccine. *Acta Trop* 111: 284–288.

[83] Wei F., Zhai Y., Jin H., Shang L., Men J., Lin J., *et al.* (2010). Development and immunogenicity of a recombinant pseudorabies virus expressing Sj26GST and SjFABP from *Schistosoma japonicum*. *Vaccine* 28:n5161–166.

[84] WHO (1965). Snail control in the Prevention of *Bilharziasis. Report of WHO Expert Committee*, Geneva, 11–214.

[85] WHO (2010). WHO Schistosomiasis Progress report 2001–2011 and strategic plan 2012–2020.

[86] WHO (2010). Intermediate hosts of Schistosomiasis and food borne trematode infections. *Freshwater Snails.* http://www.who.int/water_sanitation_health/resources/vector. Accessed 20th January, 2015.

[87] WHO (2011). *Weekly Epidemiological Record.* World Health Organisation, Geneva, Switzerland, 9: 73–80.

[88] WHO (2016a). Schistosomiasis. http://www.who.int/Schistosomiasis/en. Accessed 29th June, 2016.

[89] WHO (2016b). Schistosomiasis. http://www.who.int/mediacentre/factsheets/fs115/en/. Accessed 16th November, 2016.

[90] Wilson R.A., Li X.H., MacDonald S., Neves L.X., Vitoriano-Souza J., Leite L.C., *et al.* (2015). The schistosome esophagus is a 'hotspot' for microexon and lysosomal hydrolase gene expression: implications for blood processing. *PLoS Negl Trop Dis* 9: e0004272.

[91] Wilson R.A., Li X.H. Castro-Borges W. (2016). Do schistosome vaccine trials in mice have an intrinsic flaw that generates spurious protection data? *Parasites & Vector* 9: 89.

[92] You H., Gobert G.N., Cai P., Mou R., Nawaratna S., Fang G., *et al.* (2015). Suppression of the insulin receptors in adult *Schistosoma japonicum* impacts on parasite growth and development: further evidence of vaccine potential. *PLoS Negl Trop Dis.* 9:e0003730.

[93] You H., Gobert G.N., Duke M.G., Zhang W., Li Y., Jones M.K., *et al.* (2012). The insulin receptor is a transmission blocking veterinary vaccine target for zoonotic *Schistosoma japonicum.* Int J Parasitol 42: 801–807.

[94] You H., McManus D.P. (2015). Vaccines and diagnostics for zoonotic *Schistosomiasis japonica. Parasitology* 142. 271–289.

[95] You H., Zhang W., Jones M.K., Gobert G.N., Mulvenna J., Rees G., *et al.,* Cloning and characterisation of *Schistosoma japonicum* insulin receptors. *PLoS One* 5: e9868.

[96] Zhang W., Ahmad G., Le L., Rojo J.U., Karmakar S., Tillery K.A. (2014). Longevity of Sm-p80-specific antibody responses following vaccination with Sm-p80 vaccine in mice and baboons and transplacental transfer of Sm-p80-specific antibodies in a baboon. *Parasitology Research* 113: 2239–2250.

[97] Zhang W., Ahmad G., Torben W., Noor Z., Le L. Damian R.T. 2010. Sm-p80-based DNA vaccine provides baboons with levels of protection against *Schistosoma mansoni* infection comparable to those achieved by the irradiated cercarial vaccine. *Journal of Infectious Diseases* 20: 1105–1112.

[98] Zhang W., Li J., Duke M., Jones M.K., Kuang L. Zhang J. (2011). Inconsistent protective efficacy and marked polymorphism limits the value of *Schistosoma japonicum* tetraspanin-2 as a vaccine target. *PLoS Neglected Tropical Diseases* 5: e1166.

[99] Zhu L., Liu H.F., Lu M.B., Long Q.K., Shi Y.E., Yu L.J. (2011). Construction, purification, and evaluation of multivalent DNA vaccine against *Schistosoma japonicum. Parasitol Res* 108: 115–121.

[100] Zhu Y., Lu F., Dai Y., Wang X., Tang J., Zhao S., *et al.*, Synergistic enhancement of immunogenicity and protection in mice against *Schistosoma japonicum* with codon optimization and electroporation delivery of SjTPI DNA vaccines. *Vaccine* 28: 5347–5355.

[101] Zhu Y., Si J., Harn D.A., Xu M., Ren J., Yu C., *et al.* (2006). *Schistosoma japonicum* triose-phosphate isomerase plasmid DNA vaccine protects pigs against challenge infection. *Parasitology* 132: 67–71.

[102] Zhu Z., Fu Z., Zhang M., Han Y., Hong Y., Li D., *et al.* (2012). Protective efficacy evaluation induced by recombinant protein LHD-Sj23-GST of *Schistosoma japonicum* emulsified with three different adjuvants. Parasite Immunology 34: 341–344.

Immunomodulatory Effects of Natural Agents

Amany Sayed Maghraby* and Mahmoud Mohamed Bahgat

Department of Therapeutic chemistry, Division of Pharmaceutical and Drug Industries Research and Research Group Immune- and Bio-markers for Infection, Centre of Excellence for Advanced Science, The National Research Centre, Dokki, Giza 12311, Egypt

*E-mail: as.maghraby@nrc.sci.eg

ABSTRACT: The aim of this chapter is to review the immunoregulatory responses of natural plants, vitamins, camel milk, propolis and their potential use as adjuvants in combination with vaccines or as therapeutics. A literature search was carried out on PubMed database using the keywords propolis, Rosmarinus officinalis, vitamins, camel milk, Echinacea purpurea, Nigella sativa and Pulicaria crispia which resulted in sixty two (62) published papers over the period 1982–2018. Propolis acted as adjuvant in combination with vaccines against Gram-negative bacteria and has anti-parasitic effect. Vitamins A, E and a catechin could protect against intra-nasal challenge with live influenza virus as demonstrated by lung pathology scores, lung viral loads, and serum hemagglutination inhibition titers. R. officinalis powder and vitamin E can modulate the humoral immunity of broiler chickens. Echinacea purpurea and N. sativa combined with killed reasserted H5N1 avian influenza virus stimulated the humoral immune responses in comparison with the extract-free vaccine. N. sativa oil and its active ingredients showed Immunomodulatory activity by augmenting both natural killer cells- and T cells-mediated responses. The volatile oil of N. sativa seeds considered as a potential immunosuppressive agent. N. sativa seed oil showed potent anti-inflammatory effects on several inflammation-based models as experimental encephalomyelitis, colitis, peritonitis, oedama, and arthritis through suppressing prostaglandins and leukotriens. Methanolic extract of P. crispa reduced Schistosoma mansoni worm burden and stimulated significant IL2 as well as IgG responses that recognized bilharzial, Escherichia coli and cancer bladder antigens in S. mansoni infected mice. The beneficial effects of camel milk emanate come from their nanoparticles, especially exosomes, which were reported as anticancer agents. Some natural products have an immuno-stimulatory or suppressive response or both as propolis. The natural products can be acted as immunoadjuvants in combination with vaccines or as therapeutics to evaluate the efficacy of vaccine or drug.

Keywords: Immunomodulatory, Adjuvants, Plant extracts, Vitamins, Propolis, and Camel Milk.

1. INTRODUCTION

Under the monopoly of medicine and in light of the high costs of the pharmaceutical industry, many countries resorted to nature as a resort for treatment or to obtain pharmaceutical raw materials which can be highly economic for the African Continent (Allen 2003). Africa is rich in grasses and medicinal plants are scattered among its countries (Mousa 2017, Pleschka *et al.,* 2009). Cooperation in an integrated network might lead to self-sufficiency of natural products of medicinal or immunological values. This chapter highlights natural agents of either immune-stimulatory or suppressive responses or their potential use as adjuvant in combination with vaccines or as therapeutics.

2. MATERIALS AND METHODS

A literature search was carried out on the PubMed database using the keywords propolis, *Rosmarinus officinalis*, vitamins, camel milk, *Echinacea purpurea*, *Nigella sativa* and *Pulicaria crispia* which resulted in sixty two published papers over the period 1982-2018 (see Table 1). Propolis acted

Table 1: Summary of Immunological and Therapeutic Effects of the Reviewed Natural Agents

Natural Product	*Immunomodulatory Responses*	*References*
Propolis Water Soluble Derivative	As Anti-bacterial	Dimov *et al.*, 1992
	Klebsiella pneumoniae, Proteus vulgaris, Escherichia coli, Pseudomonas aeruginosa	
Green Propolis Phenolic Compounds	As Adjuvants	Najafi *et al.*, 2007
	Inhibitory or stimulatory Adjuvants for the growth of different cell lines	
An Ethanolic Extract of Propolis	As Vaccine Adjuvants	Fischer *et al.*, 2010
	As Vaccine Adjuvants	Ma *et al.*, 2011
		Nassar *et al.*, 2013
		Ahmed *et al.*, 2018
The Essential Oil of Brazilian Red Propolis	Anti-Parasitic	Sena-Lopes *et al.*, 2018
Vitamin E	Anti-Viral	Rehman *et al.*, 2018
Vitamins A, E and Catechin		Patel *et al.*, 2017

Natural Product	*Immunomodulatory Responses*	*References*
Echinacea purpurea	Anti-Parasitic	Allen 2003
	Anti-Viral	Mousa 2017
	As Adjuvants	Pleschka *et al.*, 2009
		Shawky *et al.*, 2015
		Razin *et al.*, 2017
Nigella sativa	Anticancer	Mollazadeh *et al.*, 2017
	Hepato-protective	Tabassum *et al.*, 2018
	As Adjuvant	Shawky *et al.*, 2015
		Soliman *et al.*, 2017
		Razin *et al.*, 2017
	Anti-bacterial	Hanafy and Hatem 1991
	Anti-inflammatory	Haq *et al.*, 1999
		Javadi *et al.*, 2018
Topical solution of Nigella sativa seed oil with honey	In wound healing of pain in rheumatoid arthritis	Mahboubi *et al.*, 2018
Nigella sativa fixed oil	Anti-fungal	Gelot *et al.*, 2012
Pulicaria crispa	Immuno-stimulatory and Anti parasitic	Maghraby *et al.*, 2010
Camel Milk	Anti-cancer	Badawy *et al.*, 2018
	Hepato-protective	Zuberu *et al.*, 2017
	Anti-parasitic	Maghraby *et al.*, 2010

as adjuvant in combination with vaccines against Gram-negative bacteria and has anti-parasitic effect. In this review, our team studied the immune-modulatory effects of *E. purpurea*, *N. sativa*, *P. crispia* on *Schistosoma mansoni* infection in mice. We also compared the immunological outcomes of mixing killed reasserted avian influenza virus with extracts of *E. purpurea* and *N. sativa* individually to those obtained by the extract-free killed virus. Moreover, we studied adjuvant effects of the same two extracts upon combination with a DNA construct encoding the HCV envelop domain in comparison to the DNA construct alone in mice.

3. RESULTS AND DISCUSSIONS

3.1 Propolis

3.1.1 *Against Gram-Negative Pathogens*

A propolis water-soluble derivative (PWSD) induced significant non-specific protection against the Gram-negative bacteria *Klebsiella pneu-*

moniae, Proteus vulgaris, Escherichia coli, Pseudomonas aeruginosa, but did not inhibit their growth *in-vitro*. Also, *in vivo* administration of the PWSD led to a rapid and route-dependent change in the alternative complement pathway haemolysis, suggesting that macrophage activation makes a major contribution to mechanism by which the PWSD prevent infections (Dimov *et al.*, 1992).

3.1.2 *As Adjuvant*

Supplementing inactivated vaccines against swine herpes virus type 1 by green propolis phenolic compounds improved both humoral and cellular responses in mice which suggests the usefulness of these compounds as adjuvants (Fischer *et al.*, 2010). Immune enhancement of propolis-derived adjuvants on inactivated porcine parvovirus vaccine in guinea pig was reported (Ma *et al.*, 2011). An ethanolic extract of propolis alone or combined with formulated inactivated *Pasteurella multocida* vaccine improved general health conditions in addition to reduction of the severity of adverse clinical signs associated with challenge infection of rabbits by *P. multocida* (Nassar *et al.*, 2013). The formulation of the attenuated *Pasteurella's* bacterin with propolis offered a potent homologous primary life-long protection to animals against infection (Ahmed *et al.*, 2018). Yang *et al.* (2015) explained a synergistic effect between Taishan *Pinus massoniana* pollen polysaccharide and propolis on enhancing immunity, which suggests that they can be used as a novel adjuvant formulation for the development of poultry vaccines as *Bordetella avium*. Co-infection of chicken by both reticuloendotheliosis virus and avian leukosis virus subgroup J suppressed immunity and resulted in vaccination failure, whereas, Taishan *Pinus massoniana* pollen polysaccharide mixed with propolis possessed an immune modulatory effect and improved the vaccination outcome (Li *et al.*, 2015).

3.1.3 *As Inhibitor or Stimulator for Growth and Proliferation Cells*

Surprisingly, in contrast to the inhibitory effect of propolis water extracts on growth of the immortalized cell lines McCoy, HeLa, SP2/0, HEp-2, and BHK21 it stimulated growth of the primary human lymphocytes in, rat's kidney, liver and spleen cells (Najafi *et al.*, 2007).

3.1.4 *As Anti-Parasitic*

The essential oil of Brazilian red Propolis is constituted of biologically active components which have both anti-parasitic and immune-stimulatory effects and can be used in the formulation of new vaccines or trichomonacidal drugs (Sena-Lopes *et al.*, 2018).

3.2 Vitamins

There is proven evidence that vitamin E possesses immunomodulatory properties that may play a positive role in disease outcomes (Bivona *et al.*, 2017). The humoral immune responses are directly affected by vitamin E, and excessive vitamin E intake has a detrimental effect on antibody production in response to naturally occurring *E. coli*, Newcastle disease virus and turkey pox vaccines both in chickens and turkeys (Friedman *et al.*, 1998). Vitamin E ameliorates brain tissue damage and alters plasma oxidative stress profiles in chickens as a result of neurotropic new castle disease virus infection (Rehman *et al.*, 2018). Also, it modulated the immunosuppressive responses of tylvalosin and florfenicol in broiler chickens (El-Ela *et al.*, 2016). Natural immune-enhancing delivery system based on the synergy of vitamins A, E and a catechin could protect against intra-nasal challenge infection with the live H1N1 2009 swine flu virus as demonstrated by reduced lung pathology scores, reduced lung viral loads, and increased serum hemagglutination inhibition titers (Patel *et al.*, 2017). Different levels of *Rosmarinus officinalis* powder and vitamin E can modulate the humoral immunity of broiler chickens, but not sufficiently to improve antibody titers against specific viral infections (Rostami *et al.*, 2018).

3.3 Echinacea Purpurea

3.3.1 *As Anti-parasitic*

Dietary supplementation with 0.1 and 0.5% ground root preparations of *E. purpurea* induced immunity following live vaccination with live Oocysts of the coccidian species *Eimeria acervulina, E. tenella, E. maxima and E. necatrix* and challenge infection with multiple avain coccidian species (Allen 2003).

3.3.2 *As Antiviral*

The frequent alterations in the antigenic structures of respiratory viruses, particularly in RNA viruses pose difficulties in the production of effective vaccines. There is scientific evidence regarding the effectiveness of several complementary therapies for cold. Thus, influenza-like illness and common cold could be treated by *Echinacea* (Mousa 2017). Along the same lines, oral zinc may reduce both duration and severity of cold. Also, probiotics exerted better effects than placebo in reducing the number episodes in acute upper respiratory tract infections.

3.3.3 *As Adjuvant*

Echinacea roots retain cytokine-modulating capabilities in an *in-vitro* human older adult model of influenza vaccination (Senchina *et al.*, 2006). Also; aerial extract alters course of influenza infection in mice through modulation of cytokines (Fusco *et al.*, 2010). *E. purpurea* extract could be a useful, readily available and affordable addition to existing control options against the avian H5N1, H7N7 and the swine-origin H1N1-S-OIV influenza viruses (Pleschka *et al.*, 2009). Extract from roots of *Echinacea angustifolia* (Polinacea) prevented respiratory tract infections and improved immune response to influenza vaccine (Di Pierro *et al.*, 2012). *E. purpurea* stimulated the response of zebrafish (*Danio rerio*) to *Flavobacterium columnare* vaccine (Guz *et al.*, 2014). Interestingly; echinacoside, a compound derived from *Echinacea* induced apoptotic cancer cell death by inhibiting the nucleotide pool sanitizing enzyme MTH1 (Dong *et al.*, 2015). Our previous work combining the HCV-E-encoding construct with extracts prepared from *E. purpurea* prior to immunizing mice increased both the humoral and the cellular (CD_4^+ and cytotoxic CD_8^+ T lymphocytes) responses compared to mice which received the DNA construct alone or PBS-treated mice (Shawky *et al.*, 2015). Also; we studied the immunomodulatory effects of a supplemented killed influenza virus (V) by *E. purpurea. N. sativa* stimulated the humoral immune responses in comparison with the extract-free vaccine which highly suggests the immune stimulatory adjuvant effect of this plant extract. The capacity of the *E. purpurea* to down-regulate both the induced cellular and humoral responses by the killed influenza virus (V) highlights the possible potential usefulness of such plant extract in supplementing vaccines prior to immunizing hyper-immune or autoimmune patients who are known to undergo severe inflammatory responses upon being vaccinated (Razin *et al.*, 2017). The prophylactic efficacy of *Echinacea* preparations, on pneumococcal and influenza vaccine was investigated. The intake of *E. purpurea* showed moderate success in preventing infection (Voß *et al.*, 2018).

3.4 Nigella Sativa

3.4.1 *As Alternative Treatment for Many Diseases*

Nigella sativa has immuno-stimulatory, anti-inflammatory, hypotensive, hepatoprotective, antioxidant, anti-cancer, hypoglycemic, anti-tussive, milk productive, uricosuric, choleretic, anti-fertility, and spasmolytic properties. *N. sativa* extracts have anticancer effects through its free radical scavenger activity and preservation of various antioxidant enzyme activities such as glutathione peroxidase, catalase, and glutathione-S-transferase (Mollazadeh *et al.,* 2017). *N. sativa* fixed oil used as alternative treatment in management of pain in rheumatoid arthritis (Mahboubi *et al.,* 2018). *N. sativa L* has a preventive role in hepatic diseases and its bioactive constituents are hepatoprotective (Tabassum *et al.,* 2018).

3.4.2 *In Wound Healing*

Javadi *et al.* (2018) demonstrated that wound healing may be improved and accelerated using topical solutions of honey, *N. sativa* seed oil and especially their mixture.

3.4.3 *Oral Health Care Products*

Spilanthes oleracea, propolis, *Nigella* seed oil, and an ethanolic extract of black garlic are promising candidates for use in oral health care products and all have the potential to control biofilm associated infections (Vlachojannis *et al.,* 2018). Fish oil/*N. sative* volatile oil emulsion was the most promising hepatoregenerative and renoprotective formula (Al-Okbi *et al.,* 2018). Thymoquinone (TQ), one of the major bioactive components of the volatile oil of *N. sativa* seed, has anti inflammatory properties by preventing the biosynthesis of mediators in inflammatory processes and asthma. TQ reduces LPS-induced proinflammatory cytokines. In addition, TQ has both cellular and humoral immunomodulatory roles (Shaterzadeh-Yazdi *et al.,* 2018). Vaillancourt *et al.* (2011) facted that TQ abolishes a number of factors known to be involved in rheumatoid arthritis pathogenesis which renders it a clinically valuable agent in the prevention of articular diseases, including rheumatoid arthritis.

3.4.4 *As Adjuvant*

A concentration of 5.6% *N. sativa* L. in broiler's feed can improve the immune response and subsequent resistance of broilers against diseases (Soliman *et al.,* 2017). Nigellone, a carbonyl polymer of TQ, isolated from *N. sativa L.* seeds. Nigellone at low concentrations is very effective in inhibiting histamine release from mast cells (Chakravarty 1993). *N. sativa* seeds contain fatty acids which completely inhibited development of Ehrlich ascites carcinoma (EAC) *in-vivo* (Salomi *et al.,* 1992). Similar work in our lab on treating mice with *N. sativa* extract prior to being immunized with a mammalian expression construct encoding the HCV envelop proteins increased both the humoral and the cellular responses compared to mice which received the DNA construct alone or PBS-treated mice

(Shawky *et al.,* 2015). Also, we showed that supplementing killed reassorted H5N1 influenza virus by *N. sativa* stimulated humoral immune responses in comparison with immunizing mice with the *N. sativa*-free killed virus which highly suggests the immune stimulatory adjuvant effect of this plant extract (Razin *et al.,* 2017).

3.4.5 *As Anti-Bacterial*

Filter paper discs impregnated in diethyl ether extract of *N. sativa* seeds (25-400 micrograms extract/disc) caused concentration-dependent inhibition of the Gram-positive bacteria *Staphylococcus aureus*, the Gram-negative bacteria *Pseudomonas aeruginosa* and *Escherichia coli* and the pathogenic yeast *Candida albicans.* The extract showed antibacterial synergism with streptomycin and gentamicin and showed additive antibacterial action with spectinomycin, erythromycin, tobramycin, doxycycline, chloramphenicol, nalidixic acid, ampicillin, lincomycin and sulphamethoxyzole-trimethoprim combination (Hanafy and Hatem 1991).

3.4.6 *As Anti-Inflammatory*

Ethanolic extract of *N. sativa L.* had a potent cytotoxic effect as well as a potentiating effect on the cellular immune response (Swamy and Tan 2000). Stimulatory response of whole *N. sativa* or fractionated proteins was noticed on the production of TNF-alpha either using non-activated or mitogen activated peripheral blood mononuclear cells (Haq *et al.,* 1999). Black seed oil proved to be an effective adjuvant for the treatment of allergic diseases (Kalus *et al.,* 2003). The volatile oil of *N. sativa* seeds could be considered as a potential immunosuppressive cytotoxic agent (Islam *et al.,* 2004). The *N. sativa* seed oil and TQ have shown potent anti-inflammatory effects on several inflammation-based models as experimental encephalomyelitis, colitis, peritonitis, oedama, and arthritis through suppression of prostaglandins and leukotriens (Salem 2005). The oil and active ingredients showed immunomodulatory activity, augmenting the T cell- and natural killer cell-mediated immune responses (Salem 2005). Importantly, the oil and its active ingredients expressed anti-microbial and anti-tumor properties against different microbes and cancers given their immunomodulatory responses (Salem 2005). Büyüköztürk *et al.* (2005) showed that *N. sativa* oil does not affect the T-helper 1 and T-helper 2 type cytokine production from splenic mononuclear cells in allergen sensitized mice. Ghonime *et al.* (2011) examined medicinal plants as *Silene nocturna, N. sativa* and *Matricaria chamomilla* growing in Egypt for their immunomodulatory effects in Balb/c mice. Immuno suppressed mice with cyclophosphamide, and pretreated with the plants extracts restored their resistance against lethal infection with the predominately granulocyte-dependent Candida albicans. *N. sativa* seed supplementation during specific immunotherapy of allergic rhinitis may be considered a potential adjuvant therapy (Işik *et al.*, 2010).

3.4.7 *As Anti-Fungal*

The oil of *N.* sativa seeds has antifungal activities (Islam *et al.*, 1989). A high antifungal activity of *N. sativa* defensins makes them promising candidates for engineering pathogen-resistant plants (Rogozhin *et al.*, 2011). Bullous drug eruption with *N. sativa* oil was studied by Gelot *et al.* (2012) where 53-year-old woman was hospitalized for febrile rash consisting of erythematous plaques with vesicles and bullous lesions and *N. sativa* oil applied to her skin. Cutaneous histopathology revealed sub-epidermal detachment and necrosis of the epidermal surface. The lesions healed slowly, depigmented macules persisted three months later. Patch tests for *N. sativa* oil were strongly positive.

3.5 Pulicaria Crispa

The plant grows in cushion shape and is widely distributed in the Mediterranean basin in Algeria, Libya, France, Syria, Palestine and Egypt. A previous report on phytochemical screening of such plant extract revealed the presence of amino acids, carbohydrates, coumarins, flavonoids, glycosides, proteins, sterols, tannins, triterpenes and volatiles. Fractionation of *P. crispa* indicated that it is rich in, flavonoids (Al-Yahya *et al.*, 1988). Immunomodulatory effects of crude extracts or purified flavonoids from plant origin as demonstrated by significant increase in IgG response against several *Schistosoma mansoni* antigens were previously reported (Shalaby *et al.*, 1999). Treating mice with methanolic extract of *P. crispa* reduces *S. mansoni* worm burden and stimulates significant IL2 as well as IgG response that recognized bilharzial, *Escherichia coli* and cancer bladder antigens. This might represent a new hopeful alternative approach for treating such diseases (Maghraby *et al.*, 2010).

3.6 Camel Milk

Camel milk ingredients including lactoferrin, immunoglobulins, lysozyme, B Vitamins, Vitamin C, minerals, and iron were studied for their medicinal properties in patients with different disorders ranging from diabetes to cancer (Rasheed 2017). Camel milk was reported to improve immunity against diseases and decrease the risk for cancer (Badawy *et al.*,

2018). Recently, most of the beneficial effects of milk come from their nanoparticles, especially exosomes, which were reported as an anticancer agent (Badawy *et al.,* 2018). Protein hydrolysate from camel milk has inhibitory effects on porcine pancreatic α-amylase, porcine pancreatic lipase and dipeptidyl peptidase-IV (Mudgil *et al.,* 2018). Camel milk exerted hepatoprotective effect in poloxamer 407 induced hyperlipidaemic wistar rats (Zuberu *et al.,* 2017). Mature camel milk has an anti-bilharzial activity in *S. mansoni* infected mice (Maghraby *et al.,* 2005).

ACKNOWLEDGEMENTS

The authors acknowledge the Egyptian Academy of Scientific Research and Technology for initiating the collaboration with The Centre for Science and Technology of the Non- Aligned and other Developing Countries (NAM S&T Centre) and the National Research Center of Egypt for approving the collaboration and for providing all logistics and facilities for preparing the chapter.

REFERENCES

[1] Ahmad, T., Rammah, S., Sheweita, S., Haroun, M. and Hamdy El-Sayed, L. (2018). The enhancement of the Pasteurella's bacterin by propolis extracts. *Rep Biochem Mol Biol* 6: 208–218.

[2] Allen, P. (2003). Dietary supplementation with Echinacea and development of immunity to challenge infection with coccidia. *Parasitol Res* 91: 74–8.

[3] Al-Okbi, S., Mohamed, D., Hamed, T., Edris, A. and Fouda, K. (2018). Hepatic regeneration and reno-protection by fish oil, *Nigella sativa* oil and combined fish oil/*Nigella sativa* volatiles in CCl_4 treated rats. *J Oleo Sci* 67: 345–353.

[4] Al Yahya, A., El-Sayed, M., Mossa, J., Kozlowski, J., Antoun, M., Ferin, M., Baird, W. and Cassady, J. (1988). Potential cancer chemopreventive and cytotoxic agents from *Pulicaria crispa*. *J Nat Prod* 51: 621–624.

[5] Ashry el, S. and Ahmad, T. (2012). The use of propolis as vaccine's adjuvant. *Vaccine* 31: 31–9.

[6] Badawy, A., El-Magd, M. and AlSadrah, S. (2018). Therapeutic effect of camel milk and its exosomes on MCF7 cells *in-vitro* and *in-vivo*. *Integr Cancer Ther* 1: 1534735418786000.

[7] Bivona, J., Patel, S. and Vajdy, M. (2017). Induction of cellular and molecular immunomodulatory pathways by vitamin E and vitamin C. *Expert Opin Biol Ther* 17: 1539–1551.

[8] Büyüköztürk, S., Gelincik, A., Ozşeker F., Genç S., Savran F., Kiran B., Yillar G., Erden, S., Aydin, F., Colakoğlu, B., Dal, M., Ozer, H. and Bilir, A. (2005). *Nigella sativa* (black seed) oil does not affect the T-helper 1 and T-helper 2 type cytokine production from splenic mononuclear cells in allergen sensitized mice. *J Ethnopharmacol* 100: 295–8.

[9] Chakravarty, N. (1993). Inhibition of histamine release from mast cells by nigellone. Ann Allergy 70: 237–42.

[10] Di Pierro, F., Rapacioli, G., Ferrara, T. and Togni, S. (2012). Use of a standardized extract from *Echinacea angustifolia* (Polinacea) for the prevention of respiratory tract infections. *Altern Med Rev* 17: 36–41.

[11] Dimov, V., Ivanovska, N., Bankova, V. and Popov, S. (1992). Immunomodulatory action of Propolis: IV. Prophylactic activity against gram-negative infections and adjuvant effect of the water-soluble derivative. *Vaccine* 10: 817–23.

[12] Dong, L., Wang, H., Niu, J., Zou, M., Wu, N., Yu, D., Wang, Y. and Zou, Z. (2015). Echinacoside induces apoptotic cancer cell death by inhibiting the nucleotide pool sanitizing enzyme MTH1. *Onco Targets Ther* 8: 3649–64.

[13] El-Ela, F., Shany, S., El-Deen, M., El-Banna, H., El-Gendy, A., Hendy, K. and Tohamy, M. (2016). Investigating the potential role of vitamin E in modulating the immunosuppressive effects of tylvalosin and florfenicol in broiler chickens. *Res Vet Sci* 108: 25–32.

[14] Fischer, G., Paulino, N., Marcucci, M., Siedler, B., Munhoz, L., Finger, P., Vargas, G., Hübner, S., Vidor, T. and Roehe, P. (2010). Green propolis phenolic compounds act as vaccine adjuvants, improving humoral and cellular responses in mice inoculated with inactivated vaccines. *Mem Inst Oswaldo Cruz* 105: 908–13.

[15] Friedman, A., Bartov, I. and Sklan, D. (1998). Humoral immune response impairment following excess vitamin E nutrition in the chick and turkey. *Poult Sci* 77: 956–62.

[16] Fusco, D., Liu, X., Savage, C., Taur, Y., Xiao, W., Kennelly, E., Yuan, J., Cassileth B., Salvatore M. and Papanicolaou G. (2010). *Echinacea purpurea* aerial extract alters course of influenza infection in mice. *Vaccine* 28: 3956–62.

[17] Gelot, P., Bara-Passot, C., Gimenez-Arnau, E., Beneton, N., Maillard, H. and Celerier, P. (2012). Bullous drug eruption with *Nigella sativa* oil. *Ann Dermatol Venereol* 139: 287–91.

[18] Ghonime, M., Eldomany, R., Abdelaziz, A. and Soliman, H. (2011). Evaluation of immunomodulatory effect of three herbal plants growing in Egypt. *Immunopharmacol Immunotoxicol* 33: 141–5.

[19] Guz, L., Puk, K., Walczak, N., Oniszczuk, T. and Oniszczuk, A. (2014). Effect of dietary supplementation with Echinacea purpurea on vaccine efficacy against infection with flavobacterium columnare in zebrafish (Danio rerio). *Pol J Vet Sci* 17: 583–6.

[20] Hanafy, M. and Hatem, M. (1991). Studies on the antimicrobial activity of *Nigella sativa* seed (black cumin). *J Ethnopharmacol* 34: 275–8.

[21] Haq, A., Lobo, P., Al-Tufail, M., Rama, N. and Al-Sedairy, S. (1999). Immunomodulatory effect of *Nigella sativa* proteins fractionated by ion exchange chromatography. *Int J Immunopharmacol* 21: 283–95.

[22] Işik, H., Cevikbaş, A., Gürer, U., Kiran, B., Uresin, Y., Rayaman, P., Rayaman, E., Gürbüz, B. and Büyüköztürk, S. (2010). Potential adjuvant effects of *Nigella sativa* seeds to improve specific immunotherapy in allergic rhinitis patients. *Med Princ Pract* 19: 206–11.

[23] Islam S., Ahsan M., Hassan C. and Malek M. (1989). Antifungal activities of the oils of *Nigella sativa* seeds. *Pak J Pharm Sci* 2: 25–8.

[24] Islam S., Begum P., Ahsan T., Huque S. and Ahsan M. (2004). Immunosuppressive and cytotoxic properties of *Nigella sativa. Phytother Res* 18: 395–8.

[25] Javadi, S., Hashemi, M., Mohammadi, Y., Mohammadi, A., Sharifi, A. and Makarchian, H. (2018). Synergistic effect of honey and *Nigella sativa* on wound healing in rats. *Acta Cir Bras* 33: 518–523.

[26] Kalus, U., Pruss, A., Bystron, J., Jurecka, M., Smekalova, A., Lichius, J. and Kiesewetter H. (2003). Effect of *Nigella sativa* (black seed) on subjective feeling in patients with allergic diseases *Phytother Res* 17:1209–14.

[27] Li, B., Wei, K., Yang, S., Yang, Y., Zhang, Y., Zhu, F., Wang, D. and Zhu, R. (2015). Immunomodulatory effects of Taishan *Pinus massoniana* pollen polysaccharide and propolis on immunosuppressed chickens. *Microb Pathog* 78: 7–13.

[28] Ma, X., Guo, Z., Shen, Z., Wang, J., Hu, Y. and Wang, D. (2011). The immune enhancement of propolis adjuvant on inactivated porcine parvovirus vaccine in guinea pig. *Cell Immunol* 270: 13–8.

[29] Maghraby, A., Mohamed, M. and Abdel Salam, A. (2005). Anti-schistosomal activity of colostral and mature camel milk on *Schistosoma mansoni* infected mice. *Asia Pac J Clin Nutr* 14: 432–438.

[30] Maghraby, A., Shalaby, N., Abd Alla, H, Ahmed, S., Khaled, H. and Bahgat, M. (2010). Immunostimulatory effects of extract of *Pulicaria crispa* before and after *Schistosoma mansoni* infection. *Acta Poloniae Pharmaceutica Drug Research* 67: 75–79.

[31] Mahboubi, M., Mohammad, L. and Mahboubi, M. (2018). *Nigella sativa* fixed oil as alternative treatment in management of pain in arthritis rheumatoid. *Phytomedicine* 15: 69–77.

[32] Mollazadeh, H., Afshari, A. and Hosseinzadeh, H. (2017). Review on the potential therapeutic roles of *Nigella sativa* in the treatment of patients with cancer: involvement of apoptosis: black cumin and cancer. *J. Pharmacopuncture* 20: 158–172.

[33] Mousa, H. (2017). Prevention and treatment of influenza, influenza-like illness, and common cold by herbal, complementary, and natural therapies. *J Evid Based Complementary Altern Med* 22: 166–174.

[34] Mudgil, P., Kamal, H., Yuen, G. and Maqsood, S. (2018). Characterization and identification of novel antidiabetic and anti-obesity peptides from camel milk protein hydrolysates. *Food Chem* 259: 46–54.

[35] Najafi, M., Vahedy, F., Seyyedin, M., Jomehzadeh, H. and Bozary, K. (2007). Effect of the water extracts of propolis on stimulation and inhibition of different cells. *Cytotechnology* 54: 49–56.

[36] Nassar S., Mohamed A., Soufy H. and Nasr S. (2013). Protective effect of Egyptian propolis against rabbit pasteurellosis. *Biomed Res Int* 2013: 1–9.

[37] Patel S., Faraj Y., Duso D., Reiley W., Karlsson E., Schultz-Cherry S. and Vajdy M. (2017). Comparative safety and efficacy profile of a novel oil in water vaccine adjuvant comprising vitamins A and E and a catechin in protective anti-influenza immunity. *Nutrients* 9: 1–17.

[38] Pleschka, S., Stein, M., Schoop, R. and Hudson, J. (2009). Anti-viral properties and mode of action of standardized *Echinacea purpurea* extract against highly pathogenic avian influenza virus (H5N1, H7N7) and swine-origin H1N1 (S-OIV). *Virol J* 6: 1–9.

[39] Razin, M., Osman, A., Ali, M., Bahgat, M. and Maghraby, A. (2017). Immune responses to killed reassorted influenza virus supplemented with natural adjuvants. *Acta Microbiol Immunol Hung* 64: 313–330.

[40] Rasheed, Z. (2017). Medicinal values of bioactive constituents of camel milk: A concise report. International Journal of Health Sciences, 11(5): 1–2.

[41] Rehman, Z., Qiu, X., Sun, Y., Liao, Y., Tan, L., Song, C., Yu, S., Ding, Z., Munir, M., Nair, V., Meng, C. and Ding, C. (2018). Vitamin E supplementation ameliorates Newcastle disease virus-induced oxidative stress and alleviates tissue damage in the brains of chickens. *Virus* 10: 173.

[42] Rehman, Z., Che, L., Ren, S., Liao, Y., Qiu, X., Yu, S., Sun, Y., Tan, L., Song, C., Liu, W., Ding,, Z., Munir, M., Nair, V., Meng, C. and Ding, C. (2018). Supplementation of vitamin E protects chickens from newcastle disease virus mediated exacerbation of intestinal oxidative stress and tissue damage. *Cell Physiol Biochem* 47: 1655–1666.

[43] Rogozhin, E., Oshchepkova, Y., Odintsova, T., Khadeeva, N., Veshkurova, O., Egorov, T., Grishin, E. and Salikhov, S. (2011). Novel antifungal defensins from *Nigella sativa* L. seeds. *Plant Physiol Biochem* 49: 131–7.

[44] Rostami, H., Seidavi, A., Dadashbeiki, M., Asadpour, Y., Simões, J., Shah, A., Laudadio, V., Losacco, C., Perillo, A. and Tufarelli, V. (2018). Supplementing dietary rosemary (*Rosmarinus officinalis* L.) powder and vitamin E in broiler chickens: evaluation of humoral immune response, lymphoid organs, and blood proteins. *Environ Sci Pollut Res Int* 25: 8836–8842.

[45] Rumjanek, M., Hanson, J. and Morly, J. (1982). Monographs in Immunology. Elsevier, Amsterdam, Sirois, pp. 267.

[46] Salem, M. (2005). Immunomodulatory and therapeutic properties of the *Nigella sativa* L. seed. *Int Immunopharmacol* 5: 1749–70.

[47] Salomi, N., Nair, S., Jayawardhanan, K., Varghese, C. and Panikkar, K. (1992). Antitumour principles from *Nigella sativa* seeds. *Cancer Lett* 63: 41–6.

[48] Sena-Lopes, Â., Bezerra, F., das Neves, R., de Pinho, R., Silva, M., Savegnago, L., Collares, T., Seixas, F., Begnini, K., Henriques, J., Ely, M., Rufatto, L., Moura, S., Barcellos, T., Padilha, F., Dellagostin, O. and Borsuk, S. (2018). Chemical composition, immunostimulatory, cytotoxic and antiparasitic activities of the essential oil from Brazilian red propolis. *PLoS One* 13: e0191797.

[49] Senchina, D., Wu, L., Flinn, G., Konopka, del N., McCoy, J., Widrlechner, M., Wurtele, E. and Kohut, M. (2006). Year-and-a-half old, dried *Echinacea* roots retain cytokine-modulating capabilities in an in vitro human older adult model of influenza vaccination. Planta Med 72: 1207–15.

[50] Shalaby, N., Maghraby, A. and El-Hagrassy, A. (1999). Effect of *Daucus carota* L.var. *boissieri* extracts on immune response of *Schistosoma mansoni* infected mice. *Folia Microbiol* 44: 441–448.

[51] Shaterzadeh-Yazdi, H., Noorbakhsh, M., Hayati, F., Samarghandian, S. and Farkhondeh, T. (2018). Immunomodulatory and anti-inflammatory effects of thymoquinone. *Cardiovasc Hematol Disord Drug Targets* 18: 52–60.

[52] Shawky, H., Maghraby, A., Solliman, D., El-Mokadem, M., Sherif, M., Arafa, A. and Bahgat, M. (2015). Expression, immunogenicity and diagnostic value of envelope proteins from an Egyptian hepatitis C virus isolate. *Arch Virol* 160: 945–58.

[53] Soliman, E., Hamad, R. and Ahmed, A. (2017). Prophylactic and immune modulatory influences of *Nigella sativa* Linn. In broilers exposed to biological challenge. *Vet World* 10: 1447–1455.

[54] Swamy, S. and Tan, K. (2000). Cytotoxic and immunopotentiating effects of ethanolic extract of *Nigella sativa* L. seeds. *J Ethnopharmacol* 70: 1–7.

[55] Tabassum, H., Ahmad, A. and Ahmad, I. (2018). *Nigella sativa* L. and its bioactive constituents as hepatoprotectant. *Curr Pharm Biotechnol* 19: 43–67.

[56] Vaillancourt, F., Silva, P., Shi, Q., Fahmi, H., Fernandes, J. and Benderdour, M. (2011). Elucidation of molecular mechanisms underlying the protective effects of thymoquinone against rheumatoid arthritis. *J Cell Biochem* 112: 107–17.

[57] Vlachojannis, C., Chrubasik-Hausmann, S., Hellwig, E., Vach, K. and Al-Ahmad, A. (2018). Activity of preparations from *Spilanthes oleracea*, propolis, *Nigella sativa*, and black garlic on different microorganisms involved in oral diseases and on total human salivary bacteria: A pilot study. *Phytother Res* 25: 1–10.

[58] Voß, S., Schnakenberg, R., Weckbecker, K. and Bleckwenn, M. (2018). Prevention of infections of the upper respiratory tract. *Laryngorhinootologie* 97: 529–536.

[59] Yang, Y., Wei, K., Yang, S., Li, B., Zhang, Y., Zhu, F., Wang, D., Chi, S., Jiang, X. and Zhu, R. (2015). Co-adjuvant effects of plant polysaccharide and propolis on chickens inoculated with *Bordetella avium* inactivated vaccine. *Avian Pathol* 44: 248–53.

[60] Zuberu, J., Saleh, M., Alhassan, A., Adamu, B., Aliyu, M. and Iliya, B. (2017). Hepatoprotective effect of camel milk on poloxame 407 induced hyperlipidaemic wistar rats. *J Med Sci* 5: 852–858.

Author Index